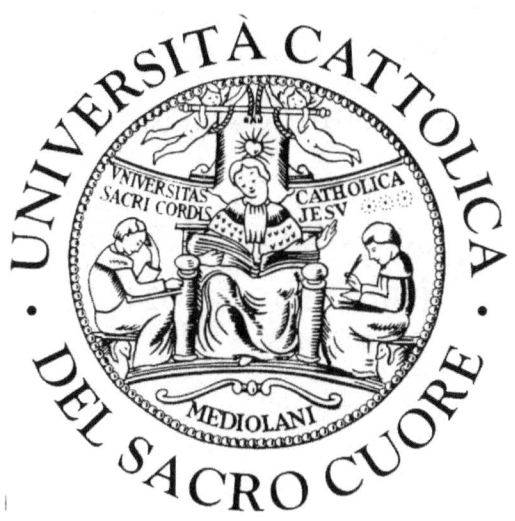

UNIVERSITÀ CATTOLICA DEL SACRO CUORE

FACOLTÀ DI MEDICINA E CHIRURGIA "A. GEMELLI"

DOTTORATO DI RICERCA IN BIOETICA

TESI

CONSCIENCE AND HEALTH CARE:
A BIOETHICAL ANALYSIS

COORDINATORE DEL DOTTORATO:

Ch.mo Prof. Antonio G. Spagnolo

Candidato:

Dott. Joseph Meaney

XXVI CICLO

CONSCIENCE AND HEALTH CARE: A BIOETHICAL ANALYSIS

Copyright © 2016 Joseph Meaney, PhD

ISBN-13: 978-1535206242
ISBN-10: 1535206241

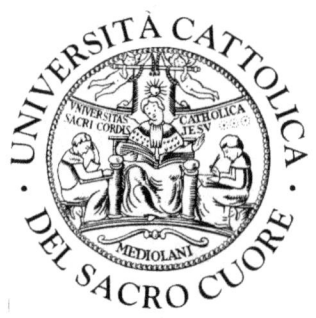

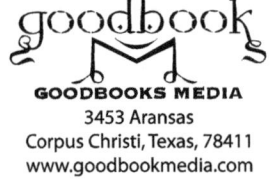

GOODBOOKS MEDIA
3453 Aransas
Corpus Christi, Texas, 78411
www.goodbookmedia.com

ACKNOWLEDGEMENTS

A project of this magnitude creates many debts and persons to whom I am grateful.

First and foremost I wish to express my deep gratitude to my wife Marie whose material and moral support were decisive in the undertaking of and conclusion of this work.

Human Life International and Msgr. Ignacio Barreiro and Fr. Shenan Boquet in particular, facilitated and encouraged my doctoral studies.

Dr. Marina Casini provided me with a wonderful example of scholarly collaboration and friendship.

Dr. Peter Saunders gave permission for and cooperated in my empirical study of the membership of the Christian Medical Fellowship UK.

My thanks go to all my professors of Bioethics, particularly my advisor Professor Antonio G. Spagnolo and Professor Adriano Pessina.

Dr. Pietro Refolo at the Institute of Bioethics provided me with useful bibliographic assistance.

I am thankful to Dr. John Haas and the National Catholic Bioethics Center for translating into English and publishing Cardinal Elio Sgreccia's *Manuale di Bioetica* which I used extensively.

Dr. Elliott Bedford very kindly sent me his dissertation on Institutional Conscience which was quite useful for my work.

Finally, and far from least, my parents, Drs. Michael & Francette Meaney, sustained and guided me with their love and example of faith and service to humanity. I will always remember and take to heart dad's insistence that what is important is God's love for us.

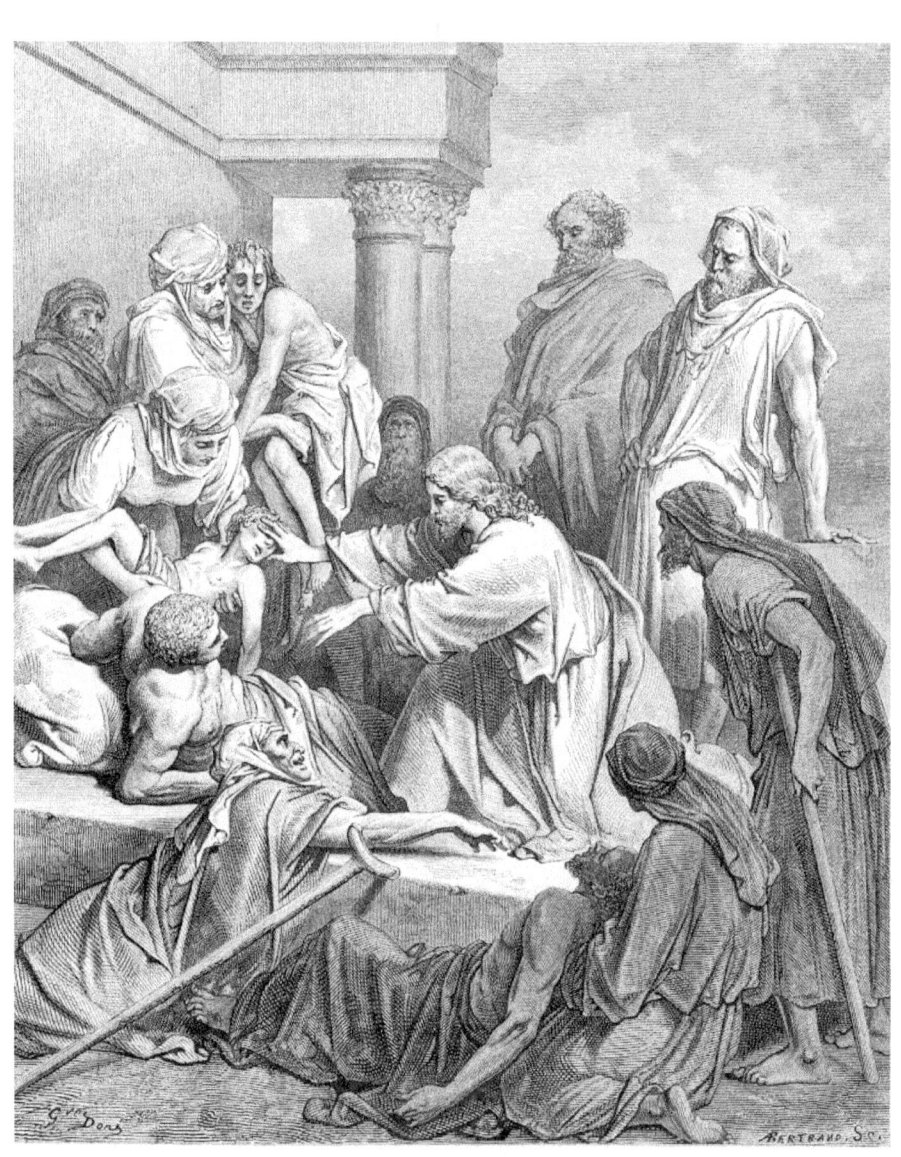

TABLE OF CONTENTS

INTRODUCTION

Writing from a scholarly, bioethical perspective on the burning ethical issue of conscience in the health care field involves many challenges. The mass media deals with this question often, but generally in a superficial and extremely polemical manner. Academic writing on the subject is also abundant. Unfortunately, many writers are not as objective in their analysis of the issues as they should be. One can detect that some authors are more motivated by the ideological clashes over abortion and other "hot button" issues such as the "morning-after pill", *in vitro* fertilization or euthanasia than by the dilemmas surrounding the application of recognized rights of conscience. Legislatures, courts, legal scholars, professional bodies, ethicists and myriad others frequently comment on this theme of conscience conflicts in health care. This means that the scholar has to sift carefully through the literature; this lengthy process of "winnowing out" the most essential contributions to the topic was a major although unseen part of the process of pulling together this dissertation.

While researching and writing, I discovered frequently a pragmatic focus among authors in the academic bioethical literature to find "acceptable compromises" for conflicts of conscience in health care. Bioethics has always been a practical and multi-disciplinary area of research, but these valuable aspects of the discipline also require a genuine investigation of the true nature of conscience rights and the logical consequences flowing from this in clinical practice. This is complicated by a glaring lack of consensus as to the exact nature of "conscience" and even as to what constitute the ends of health care. The basic need to define what conscience is escapes some authors completely with regrettable consequences. It is therefore no wonder that issues such as conscientious objection create so much division in modern, pluralistic societies.

It is my belief that an ontologically grounded personalism can make a valuable contribution and shed much-needed light on the subject of conscience in health care settings; this dissertation was written with that end in mind. Also, I share Professor Edmund Pellegrino's concern that centuries of excellent ethical reflections are, in a discriminatory manner, being increasingly marginalized simply because they stem from Catholic scholars or leaders.[1] Throughout this work, I have quoted and cited all sources that provided helpful insights

---

1 PELLEGRINO ED. *Engaging the Whole Breadth of Reason: Catholic Bioethics in the University and in the Post-Secular World* in KOTERSKI JW (editor). *Life and Learning XVIII: Proceedings of the Eighteenth University Faculty for Life Conference. Bronx:* University Faculty for Life; 2011: 3-19, p. 4.

whether from atheistic or theological perspectives. Such documents as the Christian Bible or papal declarations are therefore used, not to provide arguments from authority, but rather as historically and ethically valuable contributions to the discussion. In taking on such a broad theme as conscience and health care workers, I have had to limit the treatment of certain topics. Most importantly, I do not discuss the conscience dilemmas and rights of patients, which would be a vast undertaking in itself. One reason for this choice was the well established perception that patients' rights are currently ascendant while those of health care professionals are increasingly marginalized. I placed my main focus on the debate and situation in the United States of America (USA), although I do discuss the situation in Italy and other countries as they relate to general conscience topics and the situation of health care workers. My empirical study for this dissertation, for instance, was administered to physicians who are part of the Christian Medical Fellowship (CMF) in the United Kingdom (UK). The main reasons for focusing on the USA were that the majority of academic articles in English concern the situation there, and my own personal background, having grown up in Texas, gives me firsthand knowledge of the situation in that country.

In the first chapter, I discuss the nature of conscience. This has a historical component as the understanding of what moral conscience is has developed and changed over time. As the concept of conscience is both philosophical and theological and was greatly deepened and brought to prominence by early Christian thinkers, I pay particular attention to the Catholic tradition on the subject. In fact, the Catholic Church has developed a rich and influential understanding of conscience that is at the center of many contemporary conscience debates and is frequently opposed to secular philosophical positions on conscience in national and international fora. Also, as some modern philosophers and other thinkers, such as Friedrich Nietzsche, have taken a negative view of conscience in general, I briefly recapitulate their positions and some reasons concerning why I find their arguments unconvincing. I do the same regarding the Darwinian, Freudian and Neurological/Behaviorist approaches to conscience. Finally, I summarize why conscience is a central reality for the human person.

In chapter two, I discuss the importance of conscience as a human right. The modern era, especially from the late 18th century to the present, has focused on conscience as a basic human right. This took on a renewed impetus immediately after World War II with the Charter of the United Nations (UN) mentioning it prominently as well as that organization's Universal Declaration of Human Rights. New international law norms for what amounts to a binding obligation to refuse to violate one's conscience arose at the Nuremburg Trials, particularly the "Doctors Trials" from December 1946 to August 1947. It was a significant legal precedent in which persons, and particularly medical professionals, were for the first time condemned for not standing up to the State in defense of conscience rights.

There remains, however, a significant rift between the near universal recognition of conscience rights as human rights on a theoretical level in international fora, and widespread violations of these rights in many countries around the world. Human rights furthermore need to be grounded metaphysically, otherwise they can easily be manipulated by those wielding ideologies or their own selfish self-interest. I therefore present some of the principle theories concerning human rights, such as interest, consensus, will and social contract theory, before doing a brief investigation of the nature of the human person and the manner in which human rights are based on her human dignity. Another important topic I treat in this chapter is the hierarchy within human rights, which is a controversial topic and one with many practical consequences. I make a proposal as to how the recognition of conscience as a human right should help in the resolution of conscience conflicts involving health care workers.

Chapter three focuses on the legal and ethical dimensions of protecting conscience rights by looking at the principle strategies used to vindicate these rights. Conscientious objection, sometimes referred to as conscientious refusal, is a major issue that is treated in the academic literature. It takes the legal form of "conscience clauses" in the USA and UK, which share a Common Law system, while Civil Code countries tend to regulate conscience rights through a special "conscientious objector" status. I explain how both these systems tackle the conscience issue and their benefits as well as their limitations. Other, less frequently seen manifestations of conscience in the health care field such as civil disobedience and conscientious subversion are discussed and evaluated as well.

In chapter four, I present "special cases" regarding conscience in health care. The vast majority of writers focus on the physician, as do I in this dissertation, when discussing conscience in a medical context. Therefore, it was important to bring to light particularities that arise from the unique situations of nurses and midwives as well as pharmacists. One of the main issues regarding those major categories of health workers is an ongoing discussion regarding the "professional" standing of members of these health care specialties and if their status affects their conscience rights. Health care workers have less rights or more obligations than ordinary persons, it is often argued by bioethicists, due to their particular choice of profession and the near monopolistic nature of health care delivery. I find it unconvincing to hold either that conscience rights are reserved to certain categories of professionals or that certain categories of workers may be denied the exercise of a basic human right due to their choice of profession.

I also discuss whether health care institutions can have a conscience or whether this is limited to individuals. The existence of "institutional conscience" has been hotly challenged by some scholars in recent years even though it is in practice generally recognized and protected in conscience legislation. I pay particular attention to this concept as it has a very significant bearing on the general health care scene and how the consciences of health care workers will fare in their work environments.

Chapter five gives an overview of my empirical study of the views of physicians regarding the importance of conscience in their profession. I undertook a large study of the membership of the Christian Medical Fellowship (CMF) in the UK. With CMF's collaboration, an electronic survey on conscience and medicine was proposed to all the 2,930 practicing medical doctor members of this professional organization whose email addresses were available. The results of this study showed overwhelming support for protecting conscience rights for health care professionals consistent with other previous surveys in the UK, USA and elsewhere. It also highlighted an impression among these physicians that threats to their consciences have increased rather than decreased during their professional careers.

In the conclusion, I re-propose the personalist ethical understanding of conscience and health care. I give an overview of the topic and why health care is an activity in which protecting moral acting is particularly important. Legislative and codes of ethics protections for the conscience rights of physicians and other health care workers, and even institutions such as hospitals, are therefore vitally important safeguards and must be made more effective or increased in many instances. Unfortunately, recent years have shown an opposite trend towards the eroding of legal protections and the watering down of deontological code conscience provisions. If the exercise of conscience in health care provision is critically undermined, the remarkable power of modern advances in medicine will be increasingly placed in the hands of individuals *de facto* selected because they are willing to "obey orders" rather than stand up for their conscientious objections. The important safeguard and witness value of medical professionals with robust consciences will be removed. In a worst case scenario, the horrors of "Nazi Medicine" could be revisited with health care professionals giving in to immoral mandates in a context where medical science is many times more potent than it was in the 1930s and 1940s. It is unquestionably a grave ethical duty to promote and defend the conscience rights of health care workers committed, as Edmund Pellegrino and others stated, to the "moral enterprise" of caring for and healing the sick.[2]

---

2 PELLEGRINO ED. *The Medical Profession as a Moral Community.* Bull NY Acad Med. 1990; 66 (3): 221-232. p. 222.

CHAPTER 1:

CONSCIENCE

1.1 What is Conscience?

Moral conscience has become caricatured as the excuse and justification for almost any personal belief. Saying that my conscience compels or forbids me to do something is suspected by many as being a clever way to end all discussion or moral judgment. "It is no accident that much of our moral hand-wringing over conscience stems from its religious origins and associations and its subsequent application in a clinical, and often times secular, setting".[3] Conscience has been decried as a manipulative tool, wielded by or against the masses. Nietzsche saw conscience as the means of the weak to keep the strong in check through this powerful instrument of mind-control. Conscience is often denigrated and relegated to the Dark Ages, while at other times it is enthroned and used as excuse for any behavior and decision in our relativistic modern age. This is a deeply unfortunate development, since conscience, when rightly understood, belongs to the core of the human person, and is indispensable to her moral choices. Given the difficult ethical decisions that doctors and medical staff are confronted with every day, and the crucial role conscience plays in their professional lives, it is important to have a firm grasp on what conscience is.

Conscience, or moral conscience, is a philosophical and theological term etymologically stemming from the Latin *conscientia*, which literally means "with knowledge".[4] *Conscientia* in turn came from the Greek *syneidesis*. Both terms have a double meaning of sharing knowledge and awareness that is still present in the French *conscience*, but broken up into the two words "conscience" and "consciousness" in English.[5] Conscience is not about knowing moral evil in the abstract, but recognizing it concretely in a given case. It is a knowledge that comes before and after the choice, first warning the person that a given act or omission is morally wrong; then it is a judgment that what the person has done is condemnable, and has affected her negatively in who she is. The result of the evaluation of one's moral decisions can be a positive

---

3 HARDT JJ. *The Conscience Debate: Resources for Rapprochement from the Problem's Perceived Source.* Theor Med Bioeth. 2008; 29: 151-160, p. 152.

4 VELEZ JR. *Freedom of Conscience in Ethical Decision Making.* Linacre Q. 2009; 76 (2): 120-132, p.121.

5 LANGSTON DC. *Conscience and Other Virtues: From Bonaventure to MacIntyre.* University Park: PennState Press; 2008: p. 7-8.

one, leading to a "clear conscience", or a negative one, namely having a "guilty conscience".

It works like an inner voice, speaking with clarity and authority into one's inner core. One can try to push it to the side, attempt to drown it out, belittle the significance of what one is about to do, excuse oneself from any responsibility ("I was ordered to do it", "everybody else does it", "the hardships coming with doing the right thing were too burdensome" etc.); but it remains as a moral compass. I can even make myself sufficiently deaf to its voice, so that I eventually stop hearing it (though even then, in certain moments of crisis, I might have an awakening and hear again that long-lost call of my conscience).

Conscience is more than the abstract knowledge that, for example, stealing is wrong. I might accept that in theory, and condemn very strongly those who steal. In a situation where stealing suddenly becomes tempting, however, my conscience raises its voice and, like my better self, tells me what I should do, no matter what the costs. St. Thomas Aquinas refers to conscience as a practical act. "For conscience, according to the very nature of the word, implies the relation of knowledge to something: for conscience may be resolved into *"cum alio scientia"*, i.e. knowledge applied to an individual case".[6]

Though it is a faculty strongly related to the mind, it relates not just to my intelligence, but also to my heart and will, appealing to the best in me. It calls me from above, but fully respects my freedom in doing so. Temptation, on the other hand, appeals to my baser instincts and weak-points, trying to induce me to do something that violates what I know is right. Conscience helps me act freely and avoid subjugation to ideological demands while temptation enslaves me to whatever desires, idols, totalitarian currents to which I am willing to sacrifice my moral self.

1.1.1 Conscience in Personalist Bioethics: Its Relationship to Feelings, the Natural Law and the Truth

Throughout this dissertation, I will be referring to conscience in the following manner, as formulated by Elio Sgreccia in his book, *Personalist Bioethics: Foundations and Applications*: "The conscience can be defined as the aptitude or act of knowledge and discernment aimed at the assessment of moral actions. The conscience's object of judgment is therefore human action, which is evaluated in reference to moral values, principles, and norms. The conscience is the inner and proximate tribunal of the moral act. The truer and more comprehensive its judgment is while assessing, the more objective and valid the moral judgment will be; the more its judgment is clouded, distorted, or deprived of necessary information, the more the moral judgment could be false or erroneous".[7]

---

6 AQUINAS T. *Summa Theologica*. English Trans. FATHERS OF THE ENGLISH DOMINICAN PROVINCE. Raleigh: Hayes Barton Press; 2006: vol. I, Q. 79, A. 13, p. 746.

7 SGRECCIA E. *Personalist Bioethics Foundations and Applications*. English Trans. DI CAMILLO JA, MILLER MJ. Philadelphia: National Catholic Bioethics Center; 2012: p. 155.

Conscience is like an "inner… tribunal" in front of which a moral act is evaluated. That to which it refers for its judgment, however, must be something objective, outside of it. Otherwise, conscience would merely be a self-referential instance carrying little weight. It must therefore be pointing to an objective moral law against which it judges potential or already committed acts. This is what makes it rational and a grounded act; otherwise, it is at the whim of any desire or current fad. Truth, as expressed in an objective moral law, must therefore be its basis. As Sgreccia writes, "conscience is the rational judgment, which may be more or less systematic or intuitive, of the given value of a given act. This moral value, on the other hand, is based on ontological truth: in other words, objective truth binds reason and reason binds the conscience".[8] It is important that one explain the definition of conscience that is being used, since the discussion of conscience rights in health care can be further complicated by persons using the same word, but intending different things when referring to it.[9] It is especially true that those with a religious background and those with a secular background frequently have differing perspectives on the nature of conscience and the negative consequences of violating it.[10]

Though appealing to the heart as well as the mind, and causing feelings of guilt or contentment (when obeyed), conscience essentially involves a reasonable judgment and "is not a question of sentiment or emotion", even if these are frequently concomitant.[11] Feelings come and go; the conscience's judgment, however, stays the same (except if it was wrongly formed or blinded willfully, and is now confronted with the truth; it also becomes more fine-tuned as one becomes a better person). Feelings of guilt or satisfaction follow upon conscience's advice and our actions; they do not precede them. Because my conscience has told me that doing something is wrong, I am later haunted by regret. I wish I hadn't done it, could go back and undo the deed. Repentance and seeking to make reparation are therefore the healthy responses to a guilty conscience; they are the only way for the person to disassociate herself from the guilt she has incurred, and not let herself be determined by it forever.[12] Nevertheless, obeying the natural law for its own sake is more important than the guilt or relief we might experience in consequence, valuable as this experience might be; guilt is simply the warning signal that we have been at fault and drives us on to repent. Avoiding evil and doing the good strengthens and confirms our dignity. We are acting in accordance with the substantial orientations of our nature towards the truth and the good.

---

8 *Ibid.* p. 456.
9 LAWRENCE RE, CURLIN FA. *Clash of Definitions: Controversies About Conscience in Medicine.* Am J Bioeth. 2007; 7 (12): 10-14.
10 *Ibid.* p. 11-12.
11 SGRECCIA. *Personalist Bioethics...*, p. 155.
12 See SCHELER M. *Reue und Wiedergeburt* in SCHELER M (editor). *Vom Ewigen im Menschen.* Bern-Munich: Francke-Verlag; 1968: 27-59.

When incurring guilt and facing up to it, the person comes to realize that she has been changed through her deed or omission. What she does and says, shapes her. She may try to fool herself by asserting that everything is equal, since she has a relativistic worldview. But when she betrays, for example, a friend's confidence and, at the very latest, when that friend confronts her with it, she will probably realize that she has sinned against her friend and the trust he put in her. She has become an untrustworthy person, and the friendship may well not survive such a trial.

Our acts have consequences. Those involving a moral choice tend to carry a great weight; they shape the agent, but also the people with whom he is dealing. For example, if I neglect my child, he may well suffer all of his life from this, and do the same to his children, since abuse tends to perpetuate itself across generations. Anything I do, but in particular what I do pertaining to the moral realm, has tremendous reverberations. Treating somebody with love can help him overcome his fear and hatred of other people, and the lives of all his family may be changed. But the point here is not just that moral acts have unpredictable consequences on many lives, but that they first and foremost change us in our core, especially when it comes to serious matters.

To put this differently: when people do not show any signs of regret, or seem unaware of the enormity of their crimes, we are shocked by their moral blindness bordering on the pathological. They should feel sorry, at the very least, for having caused such suffering, even if they cannot make amends. The Nuremberg Doctor's Trials in 1946 and 1947, showed physicians and scientists who had committed crimes against humanity, but, for the most part, displayed a callous lack of regard for basic Hippocratic commandments.[13] So many defendants stated that they were just following orders, that this excuse became known as the "Nuremberg defense". Some went so far as to claim there was a general consensus in Germany that an "Order of the Führer" constituted the highest law and following these commands guaranteed the agent's innocence.[14] That they should rather have followed their conscience's dictates, when that was still lucid, did not occur to them. They were condemned by the tribunal for failing to exercise their duty to refuse to obey orders or laws that gravely violated human rights even if technically "legal" under the laws of the Third Reich. The International Law Commission stated that "the fact that a person acted pursuant to an order of his Government or of a superior d[id]… not relieve him from responsibility under international law, provided a moral choice was in fact possible to him".[15]

---

13 TAYLOR T. *Opening Statement in the Doctors Trial.* (9 December 1946). Nuremberg; 1946 (accessed on 19.09.2014, at: http://law2.umkc.edu/faculty/projects/ftrials/nuremberg/doctoropen.html).

14 WERNER B. *Affidavit.* (18 February 1947). Nuremberg; 1947 (accessed on 19.09.2014, at: http://nuremberg.law.harvard.edu/php/pflip.php?caseid=HLSL_NMT01&docnum=347&numpages=2&startpage=1&title=Affidavit..&color_setting=C).

15 INTERNATIONAL LAW COMMISSION. *Principles of International Law Recognized in the Charter of the Nürnberg Tribunal and in the Judgment of the Tribunal.* (29 July 1950). Geneva; 1950 (accessed on 19.09.2014, at: http://legal.un.org/ilc/texts/instruments/english/draft%20articles/7_1_1950.pdf).

The "Nuremberg Principles", as they came to be known, set an important precedent in international law. However, the ground on which a trial regarding crimes against humanity stands is both the assumption that there is a natural law which is accessible to everybody, and that when a positive law contradicts it in an important matter, then the first must be followed while the second must be disobeyed. These rulings must appeal to an objectively based moral conscience speaking to everyone in these situations. Conscience must be formed by the natural law and take it as its reference point; otherwise, it is in danger of becoming just as fickle as the fashion of the day.

That ethical choices shape the person one way or another becomes clear, when looking at extreme cases. Hitler and Mother Teresa, Vladimir Lenin and Maximilian Kolbe are worlds apart from each other because of the kinds of decisions they made. These are starkly contrasting examples, but they show the profound impact moral choices make on the human person. Heinous acts harden the agent to the suffering of others, particularly of his victims, while at the same time feeling self-righteous and proud to be a historical figure. Hubris makes one blind to reality, because one has first become deaf to the voice of one's conscience. Our conscience is our better self, our inner teacher, that which talks to us even when everybody else might say the contrary. It allows us to transcend ourselves and thereby fulfil our vocation as a human being, which is to seek the good and thereby grow beyond ourselves. If disregarded, we become warped by our passions, torn apart by our contradictory desires, cold-hearted to the pleas of others and tossed around by the *Zeitgeist*.

C. S. Lewis spoke about "men without chests" in *The Abolition of Man*; by denying the existence of a moral law and conscience any validity, they have lost their inner fiber, their moral core.[16] They lack the inner strength and courage it takes to do the right thing against all odds; their (even fanatic) adherence to an ideology only turns them into weather-vanes with no real backbone.[17] They have become heartless, because they have become lawless. T.S. Eliot's "hollow men" come to mind here, for they too have lost the center of their being by abandoning their sense of the good and falling into bathos and banality.[18]

1.1.2 Conscience according to the Catholic Church

For similar reasons, the Catholic Church has seen moral conscience as being of immense importance. "Conscience is the most secret core and sanctuary of a man. There he is alone with God, Whose voice echoes in his depths".[19] While every man, whether he is a believer

---

16 LEWIS CS. *The Abolition of Man*. New York: Harper Collins; 2001: p. 25-26.
17 *Ibid.*
18 SCOFIELD M. *T.S. Eliot: The Poems*. Cambridge: Cambridge University Press; 1988: p. 143.
19 PAUL VI. *Pastoral Constitution on the Church in the Modern World: Gaudium et Spes.* (7 December 1965). Rome; 1965: §16. (accessed on 17.09.2014, at:http://www.vatican.va/archive/hist_councils/ii_vatican_council/documents/vatii_ cons_19651207_gaudium-et-spes_en.html).

or not, will hear the voice of his conscience, only some will realize that this is the voice of God speaking to them. This explains why this voice speaks with such authority and that it is addressed to me, in person, as "you shall or shall not". For who but another person can address me? No thing, entity, plant or animal could do so; only a person can speak to me. For this person to be talking to me with such authority and to imply that if I do not obey, I will incur evil, that this will have consequences which I cannot, of my own accord, undo, points to the fact that the person speaking to me through my conscience is God. For who but God has the authority to do so? It must be somebody omniscient, omnipotent and all good, to know exactly what my situation is and can judge it accurately, who has the power to punish me for the evil I incur, but who wants the good and my good above all. It is along these lines that Cardinal Newman made his philosophical proof of the existence of God using conscience as his starting point.[20]

The Catechism of the Catholic Church (CCC) emphasizes the principle that, "A human being must always obey the certain judgment of his conscience".[21] This duty and right are seen as fundamental to the dignity of the human person. This spills over into civil life, so that "the Christian faithful, in common with all other men, possess the civil right not to be hindered in leading their lives in accordance with their consciences".[22] The insistence on this universal principle goes so far as to affirm that a person is obliged to follow her conscience, even if in error.[23] Why is it so fundamental to allow the subject to follow his conscience? Conscience reaches into his inner center; it is there where ultimately God enforces, encourages and warns of possible decisions, which would be evil. It would be terrible and indeed go against the dignity of the human person to prevent her from obeying her conscience. Therefore, "the Christian faithful, in common with all other men, possess the civil right not to be hindered in leading their lives in accordance with their consciences".[24]

To pressure a person to go against her conscience means demanding that she become evil; this should never be asked from another. It means dividing the person in her core, making her do something which she believes is wrong, and putting a rift between her acts and her principles. As a consequence, she has to live with a bad conscience, which will corrode her moral substance if she does not own up to it, and will set her on the wrong path. It demands

---

20 NEWMAN JH. *An Essay in Aid of a Grammar of Assent*. New York: The Catholic Publication Society; 1870. p. 60.

21 CATHOLIC CHURCH. *Catechism of the Catholic Church (CCC)*. (11 October 1992). Rome; 1992: §1800. (accessed on 17.09.2014, at: http://www.usccb.org/beliefs-and-teachings/what-webelieve/ catechism/ catechism-of-the-catholic-church/epub/index.cfm#para1768).

22 PAUL VI. *Declaration on Religious Freedom: Dignitatis Humanae*. (7 December 1965). Rome; 1965: §13. (accessed on 17.09.2014, at: http://www.vatican.va/archive/hist_councils/ii_vatican_council/documents/ vatii_ decl_19651207_dignitatis-humanae_en.html).

23 CATHOLIC CHURCH. CCC..., § 1790.

24 PAUL VI. *Dignitatis Humanae...*, § 16

of her to become, morally speaking, schizophrenic: to hold one thing right, yet act against it. Even on a natural level this cannot be good. But in the light of eternity, where our choices and who we have become determine our afterlife (except if we repent and are forgiven), it becomes all the more significant to follow one's conscience. By forcing somebody to go against his conscience, I am letting him incur moral guilt, which, especially in serious matters, might lead to his eternal death. Therefore, a person is obliged to follow her conscience, even if in error, and should be allowed to do so (in which cases she should not be permitted to do so by the State is a question I will look at in chapter three).[25]

However, this does not absolve a person from forming her conscience in light of the truth and the good. Conscience can be malformed through education, propaganda and the prevalent *Zeitgeist*. It has to be emphasized that forming one's conscience is not a private or hidden act.[26] It would be a sign of great hubris to say that I alone understand this issue and the majority are wrong, before I have done extensive soul-searching, informed myself as best I can from trusted external sources, and tried to keep an open mind. I must ask myself who the most trustworthy moral authorities in the field are as well as what great minds of integrity have thought about this. Whom do I trust among my spiritual and other mentors whose advice would be illuminating? etc.

Most importantly, one should be open to the truth and seek it with longing; for it can be difficult to discover, especially when one's own desires and the current trends are contrary to it. The knowledge that man is fallible should make him question the rectitude of his conscience, especially if it happens to be in accord with what is convenient, pleasant and in line with popular ideology. One therefore has the grave obligation to do everything possible to form one's conscience in order to make correct judgments. "Man can err in good faith with an erroneous but certain conscience. In this case the obligation remains to do everything possible—in proportion to the realities in question and in relation to one's own possibilities— so that a *certain conscience* is also true, i.e., so that the subjective judgment corresponds to objective fact".[27] The harmful objective moral content of an act committed due to an erring conscience is real and should not be taken lightly. Somebody who in good faith does something wrong and later realizes it would at least need to make amends and clearly express his sorrow for what he did, even if his responsibility was mitigated due to erroneous judgment.

There is nonetheless a grave obligation to do everything possible to form one's conscience to make correct judgments about the objective moral content of an act committed due to an erring conscience.[28] Joseph Ratzinger makes some astute points about this in his essays on

---

25 JOHN PAUL II. CCC..., § 1790. The Catholic Church, however, goes on to explain the possibility of culpability of those who follow an erroneous conscience and exhorts Catholics to form their consciences well in CCC paragraphs 1790-1794 and 1783-1785.
26 HARDT. *The Conscience Debate...*, p. 156.
27 SGRECCIA. *Personalist Bioethics...*, p. 155.
28 *Ibid.*

conscience: "Whoever equates conscience with superficial conviction identifies conscience with a pseudo-rational certainty, a certainty that in fact has been woven from self-righteousness, conformity, and lethargy".[29] What Ratzinger is getting at here is the widespread *complaisance* of people. They are convinced and strongly so, that they are right, without having thought it through, sought the truth with persistence, or realized that the truth might be contrary to their wishes. What leads to this pseudo-rational lethargy, as he explains, are self-righteousness, conformity and laziness. The first is a tremendous obstacle to a well-formed conscience since it starts with the prejudice that "I am right". How can one be open to the truth with this as a first principle? It is impossible. The combination of conformity – "everybody else is doing it so it must be right" – and laziness makes for a dangerous mixture leading to a blunted and deformed conscience, which brags of its so-called right to be the judge of things.

Furthermore, Ratzinger says that "the reduction of conscience to subjective certitude betokens at the same time a retreat from truth".[30] Over the past centuries, conscience has often been understood as something that is merely subjective which no rational argument could therefore contradict. This misunderstanding is due to a whole number of factors.

Conscience always belongs to a subject, but this does not yet make it subjective; it is simply a subject using it (an object, like a stone, could never have a conscience; only a subject can perceive, will, experience guilt etc.). Whether it is warped or false is a different question. The subject's conscience can be sound or it can be erroneous.

Saying that my conscience tells me to do something does not yet mean that I am therefore right. Perhaps some strange belief has convinced me that drowning sick children is a moral duty; if I do so, then my conscience has been distorted and my acts are objectively wrong. Conscience does not float in a neutral ethereal realm. It can be deformed and even silenced. It can only speak clearly and adequately, if it has been formed by the truth and by the good. Then it becomes a sound compass, which the person should seek to be further enlightened and formed, for example, by trusted authorities.

Unfortunately, conscience is spoken about widely today, as Ratzinger writes, as a "subjective certitude". But this subjectivity tends to take away the need to search for the truth.[31] To speak of moral conscience as detached from the truth and the good is a nonsense; by doing so, moral conscience loses both its moral authority as well as its believability. As John Paul II wrote in *Veritatis Splendor*: "Precisely for this reason conscience expresses itself in acts of 'judgment' which reflect the truth about the good, and not in arbitrary 'decisions'. The maturity and responsibility of these judgments — and, when all is said and done, of the individual who is

29 RATZINGER J. *On Conscience: Two Essays by Joseph Ratzinger*. San Francisco: Ignatius Press; 2007: p. 21.
30 *Ibid.* p. 22
31 TWOMEY DV. *Pope Benedict XVI: The Conscience of Our Age*. San Francisco: Ignatius Press; 2007: p. 124.

their subject — are not measured by the liberation of the conscience from objective truth, in favour of an alleged autonomy in personal decisions, but, on the contrary, by an insistent search for truth and by allowing oneself to be guided by that truth in one's actions".[32] Conscience without the truth and the moral law easily becomes merely the justification of our arbitrary decisions. It is no wonder therefore that it is discarded by some and instrumentalized by others. Only once one understands that conscience is ordered towards the truth and good, and that it is central to the person's moral orientation and flourishing, can one do justice to its significance, leave room even for an erroneous conscience, yet set limits to harmful excesses.

Though the State may accept some reasons for conscientious objection, even when they are far-fetched and not based on the traditional Western understanding of the moral law, it must also protect its citizens. If the moral conscience of another supposedly obliges him to perform ritual killings of human beings, then this is clearly unacceptable. A person should be prevented from doing something that is morally wrong that will hurt another, even if one must violate her conscience to do so. Personal liberties may justly be circumscribed when they affect the rights of others. The classic American legal statement of this principle is: "your right to swing your arms ends just where the other man's nose begins".[33] But this will be discussed at greater length further on.

1.2 Historical Overview

One can assume that conscience has been with humanity from the beginning. Indeed, one cannot imagine a sane person without one. Social cooperation is a human need in civilized society and would be impossible without conscience.[34] The psychopath who does not possess a sense of right and wrong does not prove this wrong, but confirms its necessity; for he is the exception to the rule. He is considered pathological precisely because he has lost his moral compass and his capacity for empathy. The scope of this thesis does not allow for an investigation as to how people become psychopaths. Suffice it to say that psychology and psychiatry confirm the importance of having a conscience by classifying those who do not as antisocial. [35]

---

32 JOHN PAUL II. *Veritatis Splendor*. (6 August 1993). Rome; 1993: §61. (accessed 18.09.2014, at: http://www. vatican.va/holy_father/john_paul_ii/encyclicals/documents/hf_jp-ii_enc_06081993_veritatissplendor_ en.html)

33 CHAFFEE Z. *Freedom of Speech in Wartime*. Harvard Law Rev. 1919; 32: 932-973, p. 957.

34 SULMASSY DP. *What is conscience and why is Respect for it so Important?* Theor Med Bioeth. 2008; 29: 135-149, p. 141.

35 HARE RD. *Without Conscience: The Disturbing World of the Psychopaths Among Us*. New York: Guilford Press; 1999: p. 76

To claim that moral conscience is an essential part of the human person in a world where evil abounds, does not mean, however, that human beings have had conceptual clarity about it from the beginning (nor do they necessarily now, for that matter).[36] *Conscientia* is an ancient Latin term used in Roman oratory well before the advent of Christianity.[37] It is derived from the Greek term *syneidesis* that also carries the double meaning of consciousness and conscience.[38]

1.2.1 Ancient Greece

In the 5th century BC, Democritus of Abdera spoke about myths regarding the afterlife as an invention of people who felt weighed down by a bad conscience. This is an early instance where *syneidesis* is referred to as moral conscience, rather than as awareness.[39]

Socrates clearly followed his conscience by choosing to die rather than admit guilt in the face of the false accusations raised against him in court. He could have escaped, as his opponents were hoping he would, but he decided that he must submit to the court, even if its verdict was unjust, to maintain his moral integrity. Already in the Gorgias, he had said: "It is a greater evil to do rather than to suffer injustice".[40] He was known to obey his daemon or inner voice in all circumstances.[41] Whether it stands for conscience or not has been much debated. The fact that it only warned Socrates regarding future decisions rather than judging past ones seems to contradict this idea, though Socrates may simply have been so obedient to his daemon, as he claims himself, that it didn't have to chide him.[42] As Linda Hogan writes in *Confronting the Truth: Conscience in the Catholic Tradition*, *syneidesis* was used in the sense of moral conscience only once by Plato. In the *Republic*, he mentions the instance of the man who is approaching death and reflects on his past conduct; as he realizes that he has

---

36 Just as the philosophical law of non-contradiction was universally used and implicitly acknowledged by people before Aristotle formulated it, so moral conscience was present and active before its more sophisticated formulations by Christian thinkers. To trace the historical development of its *prise de conscience* by thinkers does not therefore point to it being relative, as some would argue, but simply to the fact that complex data are not easily grasped and analyzed. In the moral realm, self-interest affects even the most detached person. It is understandable therefore that its objective analysis would be difficult.

37 STROHM P. *Conscience: A Very Short Introduction.* Oxford: Oxford University Press; 2011: p. 6.

38 CHADWICK H. *Some Reflections on Conscience: Greek, Jewish and Christian.* (here referred to in the German translation *Betrachtungen über das Gewissen in der griechischen, jüdischen und christlichen Tradition,* Opladen: Westdeutscher Verlag; 1974: p. 11); LANGSTON DC. *Conscience and Other Virtues...*, p. 7-8.

39 Quoted by HOGAN L. *Confronting the Truth: Conscience in the Catholic Tradition.* Mahwah: Paulist Press; 2000: p. 38-39.

40 PLATO. *Plato's Gorgias.* English Trans. JOWETT B. Rockville: Serenity Publishers LLC; 2009: p. 38.

41 ID. *Apology.* English Trans. JOWETT B. Salt Lake City: Project Gutenberg Literary Archive Foundation; 2008. (accessed on 20.11.2014, at: http://www.gutenberg.org/files/1656/1656-h/1656-h.htm).

42 HOGAN. *Confronting the Truth...*, p. 41.

committed many evil deeds, he becomes frightened. However, as Hogan also mentions, Plato and Aristotle often use the terms wisdom or prudence to speak of moral self-awareness (in ancient literature, it is generally referred to in those terms or as the heart).[43] Though they are not exactly the same as moral conscience, they overlap with some of its aspects.[44]

The Stoics believed that everybody has a divinely appointed guardian. Epictetus speaks of God handing individuals over to their conscience, once they have grown up, to guide them – a role that had been performed by a slave guarding them in childhood.[45] The Pythagoreans encouraged nightly self-examination, which is similar to the Christian examination of conscience.[46]

The term "conscience" seems to have been used widely in popular language, as Stuart Chalmers points out in his book *Conscience in Context*.[47] C.A. Pierce made a detailed analysis of the way *syneidesis* was understood in its moral meaning until the time of St. Paul.[48] In the Greek context, conscience was closely linked to *ananke* (necessity, order); thus a bad conscience was the consequence of breaking the order of the cosmos, of human nature or by going against the order instituted by the gods.[49] Furthermore, *syneidesis* always refers to the individual's acts (rather than somebody else's), specific ones at that, which are situated in the past and which are evil.

1.2.2 Ancient Rome

According to Paul Strohm in his book on conscience, the foundation of *conscientia* was originally public or social opinion; what others thought of me and of my deeds was paramount, not so much how I stood in front of my inner judge. However, the quotes he uses from Cicero suggest that public opinion and conscience are not necessarily the same, but that they should ideally be in harmony. That an orator would speak about conscience in the context of the public arena and trials makes perfect sense and does not reduce the one to the other. As Linda Hogan points out, Cicero is the first to have used conscience regularly in its exclusively moral sense. A good conscience is a blessing, while a guilty one leads to misery,

---

43 *Ibid.* p. 37-38, 40.
44 In chapter three, I will discuss briefly the reflection of moral conscience and natural law within Greek tragedy.
45 EPICTETUS. *Diss.* 111, 22, 94. Quoted by HOGAN. *Confronting the Truth…*, p. 41.
46 HOGAN. *Confronting the Truth…*, p. 42.
47 CHALMERS, S. *Conscience in Context: Historical and Existential Perspectives.* Bern: Peter Lang; 2013: p. 46.
48 PIERCE CA. *Conscience in the New Testament.* London: SCM Press; 1955: p. 40-45.
49 *Ibid.*
50 CICERO. *De Natura Deorum.* III, 85. Quoted byHOGAN. *Confronting the Truth…*, p. 42-43.

as Cicero points out repeatedly. A bad conscience is a force to reckon with, and regulates our behavior even without believing in the existence of the gods.[50]

The ancient Latin tradition is also famous for its casuistry, attempting to resolve which action to take when duties seem to conflict or the person is facing dilemmas of conscience. Cicero in particular developed a very sophisticated casuistry, looking at cases such as promising something that, as it turns out, would be harmful to the person to whom the promise has been made; or what to do after a shipwreck, when a plank can only support one person, yet a number of people are attempting to cling to it. It is interesting to see how Cicero analyzes the different circumstances carefully since this is very much in keeping with the methodology of many modern bioethicists. He writes, for example, in *De Officiis* that "different circumstances should be carefully scrutinized in every instance of duty, so that we may become skilled evaluators of duty and by calculation perceive where the weight of duty lies".[51]

1.2.3 The Bible

Conscience does not exist as a Hebrew word and is only mentioned in the Old Testament a few times when translated into Greek or in the Greek sapiential literature in the Bible like the book of Wisdom.[52] Instead, the heart is often mentioned in its stead, which includes the idea of conscience, as well as memory, volition and understanding and the whole interior life.[53] Yet without naming its reality, it is present throughout the Bible. The protagonists know when they are disobeying God's laws, and understand that they deserve punishment. If the voice of conscience is silent, for example when David commits adultery with Bathsheba, he is called back to his senses by the prophet, Nathan. Pedagogically astute, Nathan uses another example, analogous to David's sin, to make the king condemn the rich owner who steals the only sheep of his neighbor, thereby judging himself. Once David recognizes the gravity of his sin in having seduced Uriah's wife and then sending him to his death to cover up his own guilt, he puts on sack-cloth and ashes to do penance.[54] The term "conscience" may not be present in the text, but Nathan has clearly awoken his conscience, which condemns him and urges him to do penance.

---

51 CICERO. *De Officiis* 1, 32. Quoted by HOGAN. *Confronting the Truth...*, p. 45.

52 As Hogan points out, the term "conscience" only appears explicitly two or three times in the Old Testament. For example, in the book of Wisdom (Wisdom 17:11) and in Psalm 139 (Psalm 139:1 23-4). Self-knowledge arises through God revealing Himself and the law; through this the person knows if she lives in accordance with what is right. She must not only obey the law, however, but let her heart be transformed by it. HOGAN. *Confronting the Truth...*, p. 46-7. See also CHALMERS. *Conscience in Context...*, p. 63.

53 JAGER E. *The Book of the Heart.* Chicago: University of Chicago Press; 2000: p. 10. See also ANDREW EG. *Conscience and its Critics: Protestant Conscience, Enlightenment Reason, and Modern Subjectivity.* Toronto: University of Toronto Press; 2001: p. 12. The equivalent to conscience in the Old Testament is heart ("leb").

54 Though he does so only while his son is alive in the hope of swaying God's punishment, he is still making penance for a sin he clearly recognizes.

Already at the very beginning of the Bible, Eve's conscience comes to the fore, it seems, when she first withstands the serpent's suggestion to disobey God. She repeats to him God's prohibition, thereby correcting the serpent who insinuates that God is a tyrant and a liar. Once she and Adam have eaten from the forbidden fruit, however, their bad conscience becomes apparent. They hide from Him, are fearful and ashamed, and God punishes them for their sin. Later when Cain thinks of killing his brother Abel, God challenges him, asking him why he is angry. He warns him that sin is lurking: "Then the Lord said to Cain: Why are you angry? Why are you dejected? If you act rightly, you will be accepted; but if not, sin lies in wait at the door: its urge is for you, yet you can rule over it".[55] God wants to alert Cain to the fact that he is close to committing sin, but that there is still time to turn back. After the murder, God asks Cain where his brother is. When Cain doesn't want to give a straight answer, God says: "What have you done? Your brother's blood cries out to me from the ground"![56] There are many instances of a bad conscience in the Old Testament, which we need not list exhaustively for our purposes. The only time conscience is explicitly mentioned in the gospels, is when the woman is caught in adultery. The crowd who wanted to stone her leaves one by one "convicted by their conscience".[57]

Saint Paul, however, is the main biblical source about conscience. He uses the term *syneidesis*, in his letter to the Romans. "For when the Gentiles who do not have the law by nature observe the prescriptions of the law, they are a law for themselves even though they do not have the law. They show that the demands of the law are written in their hearts, while their conscience also bears witness and their conflicting thoughts accuse or even defend them on the day when, according to my gospel, God will judge people's hidden works through Christ Jesus".[58] It seems that there was no philosophical awareness of conscience as a concept before Paul; it was only used, according to Chadwick, in popular language.[59] Paul takes it over from the Greeks, but develops it further.[60] He speaks about the law written on everyone's hearts, even the pagans'; thus even without the explicit, positive law of God given through the Ten Commandments and not knowing Christ's teachings, they are still without excuse if they sin. For they know the moral law which is inscribed on their hearts, as Paul writes. He uses the heart as a metaphor for "divine law, conscience, and the incarnated Gospel", as Eric Jager points out.[61] Conscience

---

55 The Holy Bible. New American Bible Revised Edition. Washington, DC: Fairbrother; 2011: Genesis 4:7-8. (accessed 17.09.2014, at: http://usccb.org/bible/genesis/4).
56 *Ibid.* p. 10
57 JOHN 8: 9.
58 ROMANS 2: 14-15.
59 CHADWICK. *Some Reflections...*, p. 11-12.
60 CHALMERS, *Conscience in Context...*, p. 43-44.
61 JAGER. *The Book of the Heart...*, p. 10. He also points out that Paul speaks about the "tablet of the heart" as the divine law written in people rather than the tablets of stone, on which Moses wrote the ten commandments.

is this intuitive knowledge of the natural law, as it arises in particular circumstances; it guides and warns before, and condemns after the deed.[62] Yet it is not infallible and is separate in Paul's understanding from God's judgment.[63]

Christianity took on the Latin term of consciencia, when Jerome translated the Bible from Greek into Latin and chose this term to render the Greek syneidesis in Paul's letter.[64] The latter, according to Strohm, has a more inward-looking quality, while consciencia also looks outwardly to public opinion and shared values.[65] I would disagree with Strohm here, for consciencia, at least in its Christian understanding, looks to the unchangeable, natural law inscribed in the human heart as it is also expressed (hopefully) within public mores and the law. However, when the legal system or the common values contradict the natural law, then the well-formed conscience has to turn against the Zeitgeist and follow the dictates of absolute moral norms.

An example of the law also being inscribed on the Gentiles' hearts and conscience beckoning them to act rightly, is dramatically shown in Pontius Pilate's case. He knows Christ is innocent, tries to save him, but will not risk his own career and life to do so. Christ holds him responsible for his deed, though he says that the one who betrayed him is more at fault.[66] Christ does not let him off the hook lightly; he is responsible for what he is doing, for he knows that Christ is innocent and only caves in to the pressure and blackmail from the crowd.[67]

1.2.4 Theologians

The early Church Fathers, particularly St. Clement I, St. Ignatius of Antioch, St. John Chrysostom and Tertullian wrote often about conscience.[68] In his Confessions, St. Augustine speaks about conscience and the way it admonishes and urges him, even "gnawing" within him, putting him to shame before his conversion.[69] He knew at a certain point that Manichaeism was wrong, and that Christianity was right, having listened to St. Ambrose's sermons and argued with his friends, many of whom had already converted. Yet, he cannot make the step, mainly because he does not want to embrace chastity. His conscience speaks

---

62 *Ibid.* p. 17.
63 CHALMERS. *Conscience in Context…*, p. 57-58.
64 LANGSTON. *Conscience and Other Virtues…*, p. 9.
65 STROHM. *Conscience…*, p. 8.
66 JOHN 19: 11.
67 MATTHEW 27: 22-26.
68 ASHLEY B. *Elements of a Catholic Conscience* in SMITH RE (editor). *Catholic Conscience: Foundation and Formation: Proceedings of the Tenth Bishops' Workshop*, Dallas, Texas. Braintree: The Pope John XXIII Medical-Moral Research and Education Center; 1991: 39-57, p. 44.
69 AUGUSTINE. *Confessions of Saint Augustine*. English Trans. SHEED FJ. London: Sheed & Ward; 1984: p. 134.
70 *Ibid.*

to him, "indeed you kept saying how that you would not cast off the burden of vanity for an uncertain truth" and yet he does not make the step.[70] Conscience, as Strohm points out, "speaks from a position shared with the self, but incorporates elements and perspectives external to the self".[71] It speaks from within one's heart, yet it expresses itself with a knowledge and authority going beyond the self.

In the Middle Ages, conscience was further analyzed and fleshed out. The Church was the chief moral authority in Western Europe, and strengthened the role of conscience, the content of which was not easily doubted. In Peter Celle's allegory *On Conscience* from the 12th century, conscience arrives like a queen to the banquet, carrying cases of scrolls that specify its contents.[72] There is no ambiguity, no question about the reference-point of conscience. In the medieval English classic *Ayenbite of Inwyt* ("Repeated Gnawing of Conscience") from the mid-14th century (the French original was from the 13th), the Christian can measure his actions against the doctrine of the Church, the seven deadly sins, God's commandments, the cardinal virtues etc.[73]

Much of the medieval discussion on conscience was centered on the distinction between *consciencia* (or *syneidesis*) and *synderesis*. This distinction came about because of what was probably a transcription error of Jerome in his *Commentary on Ezekiel*.[74] *Syneidesis* was thought to refer to particular judgments of conscience, while *synderesis* was supposed to mean the "spark of conscience" or the general orientation towards the good.[75] St. Thomas Aquinas was the most important Scholastic writer on conscience. He saw *synderesis* as part of human nature, a habit of practical reason, intuitively grasping the primary principles of action, as he explains in the *Pars Prima* of the *Summa Theologica*, while *consciencia* applies these first principles to particular situations.[76]

At the time, there had been a wide range of opinions on the question whether the judgments of conscience were binding or not. St. Augustine thought conscience never was, except as God's delegate, which was the widespread opinion of his day. Aquinas, following Albert the Great, believed it always was binding, to the point that the subject must even obey an erroneous conscience.[77] In one of his first works, the *Commentary on the Sentences*, Aquinas

---

71 STROHM. *Conscience...*, p. 8.

72 *Ibid.* p.12.

73 *Ibid.*

74 VISCHER RK. *Conscience and the Common Good: Reclaiming the Space between Person and the State.* Cambridge: Cambridge University Press; 2010: p. 52.

75 HOGAN. *Confronting the Truth...*, p. 59-60, 66-67.

76 *Ibid.* p. 76-77.

77 As mentioned earlier, his has become the official teaching of the Catholic Church. "A human being must always obey the certain judgment of his conscience. If he were deliberately to act against it, he would condemn himself. Yet it can happen that moral conscience remains in ignorance and makes erroneous judgments about acts to be performed or already committed". CATHOLIC CHURCH. CCC..., § 1790.

argued that it would be wrong to go against one's conscience, since it is compulsory – whether it is right or wrong. In the case of conscience being in conflict with divine law, Aquinas says in *De Veritate* that one is only bound by a law that one knows; this led him to conclude in the *Summa* that the man not capable of knowing a law is not bound by it or only insofar as he should have known about it.[78]

Thomas Aquinas followed St Paul in recognizing the possibility of an erroneous conscience that one would have to obey to avoid incurring guilt.[79] The Catholic Church allows for the concept of "invincible ignorance", that somebody through no fault of his own is doing serious evil without realizing it. Aquinas' conclusion was not to "act according to your conscience", however, but rather to "inform your conscience objectively, and then act according to it".[80] For human beings have the duty to form their consciences by turning to sources of truth and authority, like the Church, that will give them clear guidance. To say, "I didn't know", is not good enough, if the person did not truly and diligently seek to discover what is right and what is wrong.

Obedience to the Catholic Church was rejected by the Protestant Reformation. The Reformers accepted as guides for the person's conscience only the Holy Spirit and the Bible that depended on her personal, albeit divinely inspired, interpretation. God was understood as communicating directly with the soul through the Bible. In his declaration of Worms from 1521, Martin Luther declared: "I cannot and I will not recant anything for to go against conscience is neither right nor safe".[81] Johann Eck, who was secretary to the proceedings, then called out to him to lay aside his conscience, "because it is in error".[82] In 1525, Luther would write in his work "On the Bondage of the Will", that "consciences are bound only by a commandment of God, so that the interfering tyranny of the popes… has simply no place in our midst".[83]

---

78 HOGAN. *Confronting the Truth…*, p. 81-84.
79 In his first Letter to the Corinthians, Paul allows for an erroneous conscience that must nonetheless be obeyed. CHALMERS. *Conscience in Context…*, p. 58-59; HOGAN. *Confronting the Truth…*, p. 52-53.
80 ASHLEY. *Elements of a…*, p. 45.
81 Quoted in VISCHER. *Conscience and the Common Good…*, p. 56.
82 STROHM. *Conscience…*, p. 24.
83 *Ibid.* p. 25.
84 As John Haas points out in his article "Crisis of Conscience and Culture", there are various elements of Protestantism which have undermined the understanding of conscience as a reliable guide (albeit in need of formation and guidance). Human nature and reason itself are thought to be completely corrupted. Hence, conscience ultimately cannot be trusted. Furthermore, if one is saved by grace alone, then it does not matter if one sins or not. One can, as Luther said, "sin boldly". *Sola scriptura, sola gratia, sola fides* and the individual as *simul justus et peccator* have all contributed to the individualistic manner in which conscience has been understood in modernity. HAAS J. *Crisis of Conscience and Culture* in HAAS J (editor). *Crisis of Culture*. New York: Crossroad; 1996: 21-47, p. 30-32.

Yet this faith in an infallible conscience did not last long, and soon conscience was seen as prone to delusion since it too was wounded by the Fall.[84] Calvin, for example, thought that it was in need of healing by God, since it otherwise would tremble in fear in front of God's wrath. Faith became the guarantor of salvation rather than conscience viewed as too timorous to take on that role.[85]

1.2.5 Secular Thinkers

The separation of conscience from the Church and religion could therefore arguably be seen to originate in the Reformation rather than in the Enlightenment, as Strohm points out.[86] Interestingly, it is in consequence of the conflicts generated by the various religious denominations, that the modern notion of freedom of conscience as a human right was developed by John Locke. In his *Letter Concerning Toleration* (1689), he bases his argument for religious freedom upon the idea of human rights. His hope is that churches would "lay down toleration as the foundation of their own liberty, and teach that liberty of conscience is every man's natural right".[87] Civil as well as religious authority should respect religious practice as belonging to the realm of conscience. He tries to develop a structure allowing for the use of conscience within a realm governed by civil law. In his *Essay Concerning Human Understanding* (1690), Locke states that conscience should be governed by human reason; it is neither innate nor the result of divine inspiration. People's consciences lead them to do contradictory things; what is considered good by one may be thought to be evil by another. Hence, conviction and enthusiasm are not sufficient to evaluate somebody's conscientious decision; instead, reason must do so. Custom and consensus are important factors as well, according to Locke since he sees conscience as being formed through experience.[88] But against what can customs and consensus be measured, is a question that needs to be raised. What must reason follow in order to be reasonable? It seems that only an objective moral order can serve as such a measuring rod.

Within the 18th century, the emphasis regarding moral choices was put increasingly on reason, but also on feeling. The problem with these approaches was their circularity as well as their lack of objectivity. Without external authority, reason is in danger of falling into error or being led astray by personal self-interest. Since the authority of a Church, the idea of an interventionist God and of an objective natural law were increasingly repudiated, one had to turn towards consensus and social norms to evaluate moral action.

Immanuel Kant in his *Grounding of a Metaphysics of Morals* therefore came up with the

---

85 STROHM. *Conscience…*, p. 27-29, 37.
86 *Ibid.* p. 37-38.
87 LOCKE J. *A Letter Concerning Toleration.Minneapolis*: Filiquarian Publishing LLC; 2007: p. 51.
88 This view is quite influential today. VISCHER. *Conscience and the Common Good…*, p. 60.

idea of a moral law that is universal, because each time I act, I must ascertain if this action is applicable to everybody else. Hence, any action pertaining to the moral realm must be universally valid or I had better abstain from it.[89]

The problem with the Enlightenment's emphasis on consensus as a reference point for conscience, was that it left the individual at the mercy of the *Zeitgeist*, of being easily swayed by public opinion and of later being at the mercy of totalitarian regimes that could impose their ideology on everybody. How is the individual to stand against such forces, if consensus is the ultimate reference-point for conscience?

To counteract such tendencies, the utilitarian philosopher, John Stuart Mill, who influenced substantially the modern understanding of religious and political liberties, fought for tolerance and the rights of the minority against the majority. It is to him that we owe the widespread idea that the protections for individual autonomy and action stop where these start harming someone else, as he expounded in his *Essay on Liberty* (1859). He criticized the "despotism of custom" and of collective opinion.[90] Many of those in the 20th century who spoke of a right to conscientious objection harkened back to Mill's philosophy.

1.2.6 John Henry Newman

With John Henry Newman, we find a thinker who brought conscience to new prominence. He states that the reasons for contradictory theories regarding conscience are due to two fundamental ways of seeing conscience, namely as a mere matter of taste or as the "echo of the voice of God".[91] In his *Letter to the Duke of Norfolk*, he states that instead of understanding conscience as a duty towards God, it is now widely used as excuse for self-will and personal preference.[92] As Hermann Geissler writes in his article "Truth and Conscience in the Writings of Blessed John Henry Newman", "for him, conscience is not an autonomous but a fundamentally theonomous reality – a sanctuary by which God turns intimately and personally to every soul".[93] In that same letter, Newman writes beautifully about conscience being a "messenger from Him, who, both in nature and in grace, speaks to us behind a veil, and teaches and rules us by His representatives. Conscience is the aboriginal Vicar of Christ,

---

89 In his *Metaphysics of Morals*, Kant speaks of conscience as an "internal court in man", and about the problem that one instance cannot be prosecutor, jury and judge at the same time without conflict of interest. Hence, the individual must think about himself as another person in order to assess himself objectively. God thereby becomes a subjective principle, somebody I imagine judging myself, but remaining a part of my own being. STROHM. *Conscience...*, p. 45-46.

90 MILL JS. *On Liberty.* London: Longmans, Green, and Company; 1921: p. 41.

91 NEWMAN JH. *Sermon Notes.* Notre Dame: 2000; p. 327. Quoted in GEISSLER H. *Conscience and Truth in the Writings of Blessed John Henry Newman.* (accessed on 04.10.2014, at: http://www.newmanfriendsinternational. org/newman/wp-content/uploads/2013/05/conscience-and-truthin- the-writings-of-blessed-jhn.pdf).

92 NEWMAN JH. *Diff II...*, p. 250

93 GEISSLER. *Conscience...*, p. 8.

94 NEWMAN. Diff II..., p. 248.

a prophet in its informations, a monarch in its peremptoriness, a priest in its blessings and anathemas…".[94] Conscience is therefore at the very core of moral life and of the person's relationship to God.

In his *An Essay in Aid of a Grammar of Assent* (1870), Newman tries to prove the existence of God by taking conscience as his point of departure.[95] He distinguishes between the moral sense and the sense of duty; the first is reason grasping which action is right and which is wrong, while the sense of duty confronts us with a command that we must obey. Who can address us with a moral command that bears such authority other than an absolutely good and just God? The consequences of obedience or disobedience are the emotions we know: serenity, peace and happiness in the first case, shame, fear and guilt in the second. This is also why, according to him, conscience "is always emotional".[96] We feel emotions *vis-à-vis* persons, but not in front of animals, objects, laws etc. So the fact that we feel remorse, fear and sorrow, when committing evil, points to the fact that we have sinned *vis-à-vis* a person with the authority to judge us.[97] Though Newman did not discard the traditional proofs of God's existence, he preferred his path, since it starts with the person's experience of interiority and leads to the encounter with a personal God rather than with a prime cause.[98] In conscience, God interacts with the individual, guiding, warning, and reprimanding him.

In his *Dispositions for Faith* (1856), Newman addresses the issue that conscience is sometimes unclear; one must be attuned and open to the truth to hear it clearly and follow its every prompting.[99] Paradoxically, it is commanding, yet soft-spoken at the same time. Hence, the desire arises in those who are ethically awake to gain greater clarity, and to be sure of doing the right thing. It therefore predisposes the person, as Newman writes, for revelation. "So the gift of conscience raises a desire for what it does not itself fully supply. It inspires in them the idea of authoritative guidance, of a divine law; and the desire of possessing it in its fulness (sic), not in mere fragmentary portions or indirect suggestions".[100] A person who has a fine-tuned conscience will therefore seek greater clarity, try to explore in depth what to do in morally complex situations and seek the truth rather than use the easy excuse of his

---

94 Id. *An Essay in Aid of…*, p. 60.

95 Id. *An Essay in Aid of…*, p. 60.

96 Quoted by IGLESIAS ROZAS T. *Newman on Conscience and our Culture*. Milltown Studies. 2002; 49: 19-49, p. 37; NEWMAN JH. *An Essay in Aid of a Grammar of Assent*. KER I. ed. Oxford: Clarendon Press; 1985.

97 ROZAS. *Newman on Conscience…*, p. 40-41.

98 GEISSLER. *Conscience…*, p.10.

99 NEWMAN JH. *Sermons Preached on Various Occasions*. London: Longmans, Green, and Co.; 1908: p. 69.

100 *Ibid.* p. 66.

101 Professor Robert George emphasizes this point with reference to Newman's thought. Conscience is a "stern monitor" not a "writer of permission slips" and conscience imposes duties and obligations rather than allowing one to do as one pleases. GEORGE RP. *Conscience and its Reviewers: A Response to Kevin Doyle* (20 November 2013). Princeton; 2013 (accessed 17.11.2014, at: http://www.thepublicdiscourse.com/2013/11/11233/)

102 ID. *Conscience and its Enemies: Confronting the Dogmas of Liberal Secularism*. Wilmington: ISI Books; 2013: p.112.

conscience prompting him to do something that coincides with his liking and that he has not taken the trouble to question.[101] Newman speaks of conscience as something like the opposite of "autonomy in the modern liberal sense" because it imposes concrete obligations and duties rather than giving a license to do as one pleases.[102]

1.3 Selection of Main Modern Arguments Against Conscience

1.3.1 Nietzsche

There are a number of standard approaches taken regarding the concept of conscience. One is to hold that conscience is a construct put into place by the weak to protect themselves against the stronger. In his book, On the Genealogy of Morality (1887), Nietzsche defends the idea that the good was originally what the nobility embodied, namely power, vitality, nonchalance, confidence, truthfulness, spontaneity etc., while the bad was what the common man stood for, i.e. weakness, cowardice and misery.[103] Since the weak could not stand the superiority of the powerful, they got the better of them by bringing about a revolution of morality.[104] While power had previously been deemed something good, it was now considered evil, while weakness, sickness and cowardice were now esteemed highly. This reversal of values, which Nietzsche calls the slaves' revolt in morality, was brought about through Christianity, he claims. It was fuelled by resentment, at the root of which lies anger that cannot express itself directly, since the angry person is not strong enough to stand up against the other. The weak individual therefore compensates for his inferiority through imaginary revenge, or by bringing down the other through indirect means.[105] Since the strong were no longer allowed to express their power through violence after the advent of Christianity, *dixit* Nietzsche, they were obliged to turn their aggressions inwards and torment themselves by means of a bad conscience. Conscience was invented, so that the strong would "hurt himself after the more natural vent to his desire had been blocked".[106] In the section, 'Why I write such Excellent Books', in *Ecce Homo*, Nietzsche states that conscience "is not, as you may believe, 'the voice of God in man'; it is the instinct of cruelty, which turns inwards once it is unable to discharge itself outwardly".[107]

I need not criticize every aspect of Nietzsche's theory for my purposes here. What his

---

103 NIETZSCHE F. *On the Genealogy of Morals: A Polemical Tract*. English Trans. JOHNSTON I. Arlington: Richer Resources Publications; 2009 (accessed 17.11.2014, at: http://home.sandiego.edu/~janderso/360/genealogy2.htm).
104 *Ibid.* No.15-16.
105 *Ibid.* No. 20-21.
106 Quoted in STROHM. *Conscience...*, p. 65.
107 *Ibid.* p. 69.

philosophy and values lead to was shown by the Third Reich. But let us envisage a toned down version of Nietzsche's theory which is still very much alive today, namely that conscience is merely a construct. Underlying it – like every other theory denying the validity of conscience as our moral compass – is the relativity of good and evil. The one flows logically from the other; if good and evil are not absolute realities, then neither will conscience's unconditional "no" to some things be an indicator of an objective moral law.[108]

The example of extreme evil shows most clearly that evil is not relative, and the reductionist theory that good is nothing but self-interest is not convincing either. For not only were the victims of the Holocaust or under other totalitarian regimes absolutely certain about the existence of objective evil as it was being done to them, but so were those onlookers who were not blinded by ideology, fear or self-interest. Somebody like Oskar Schindler was out for his own profit at first, but when he finally realized the humanity and dignity of the Jews, he tried to save as many as he could, even though it went against his own financial interest. His good deeds contradicted his self-interest, which indicates that the two are not the same.[109]

Those who commit evil while self-deluded into believing there is no evil, often find themselves guilt-ridden despite their convictions. This is a common experience which has been captured in many novels and movies. Since good and evil are basic realities, as I would claim, one cannot prove their existence by going back to something that would precede them. This would mean reducing them to something they are precisely not, like saying that good is nothing but my self-interest. When looking at the good and self-interest separately, however, one can see where they differ. The good may well be calling me to do something, which goes against my self-interest (like visiting a sick acquaintance while I would much rather take a nap); it is tempting to follow my own selfish desires, but when I don't, I know that I am doing the right thing. It is a fallacy to think that by reducing something to what is lower, one is doing it justice and understanding it better. Something that is *sui generis*, of its own kind, can only be understood in its own right.

Going back to Nietzsche's idea that conscience is a construct used to hold the stronger in check, one has to see it for what it is: a hypothesis. To say that it is the product of resentment, a clever manipulative tool, fails to do justice to the fact that conscience is reflected in ancient literature, as I have shown earlier on, even though it took centuries and Christianity to bring it to greater philosophical clarity. Furthermore, to hold that Christianity is merely the outgrowth

---

108 The problem with proclaiming the relativity of good and evil is that it cannot be held without contradicting oneself through one's very acts. As C.S. Lewis puts it in *Mere Christianity*, the greatest relativist will blow his theory to the winds, when an injustice is being done to him. While relativism can be a very pleasant and practical position allowing one to act as one pleases, it has the unfortunate shortcoming that it will permit others to do just the same. LEWIS CS. *Mere Christianity*. London: Collins; 1988: p. 6.

109 The fact that the good always has positive effects on the soul still does not make it the same as self-interest. If I do the good merely for my own sake, it hollows it out so to speak and the good effects on me are largely negated.

of resentment shows a complete misunderstanding of the reality and views of this religion. Weakness and misery are not seen as goods in the Christian vision; instead, Christians combat these evils by assisting the poor and needy, and have throughout the history of the Church. Health and strength are perceived as valuable, but not as absolute goods, for they can be used to do evil.

1.3.2 The Darwinian Approach

Another variant of the idea that conscience is simply a construct would be to say that conscience is part of the Darwinian process to keep society ordered, that it had its place and perhaps still has, but that it eventually can be discarded. Not surprisingly, Richard Dawkins writes in *The God Delusion*, that our understanding of right and wrong is an artefact of our evolutionary history.[110] Charles Lineweaver argues that conscience has evolved just like other features such as skin color.[111]

In his book *The Descent of Man*, Darwin speaks about the evolution of morality from social qualities which had been acquired through natural selection.[112] He affirms that the moral sense or conscience is by far the most important difference between man and the lower animals and the noblest attribute of man.[113] Nevertheless, natural selection explains the existence of different moral systems which cannot be judged in terms of their moral content, but only insofar as they promote the survival of the fittest in his view. Conscience is a feeling of unease or dissatisfaction which invariably results from any unsatisfied instinct.[114] Darwin was, in keeping with his theories, against the civilizing tendencies of caring for the sick and needy who should rather be left to die. "We civilized men, on the other hand, do our utmost to check the process of elimination; we build asylums for the imbecile, the maimed, and the sick; we institute poor laws; and our medical men exert their utmost skill to save the life of everyone to the last moment. There is reason to believe that vaccination has preserved thousands, who from a weak constitution would have formerly succumbed to small-pox. Thus the weak members of civilized societies propagate their kind. No one who has attended to the breeding of domestic animals will doubt that this must be highly injurious to the race of man".[115] Such shocking words clearly show, as Wike in his article "Darwin and the Descent of Morality" concludes, that Darwin was the first social Darwinist despite modern attempts

---

110 DAWKINS R. *The God Delusion*. London: Bantam Press; 2006: p. 241ff.
111 LINEWEAVER CH. *Increasingly Overlapping Magisteria of Science and Religion* in GORDON R, SECKBACH J (editors). *Divine Action and Natural Selection: Questions of Science and Faith in Biological Evolution*. Singapore:World Scientific; 2008: 171-181. p. 174.
112 Quoted by WIKE B. *Darwin and the Descent of Morality*. First Things. November 2001 (accessed on 17.11.2014, at: http://www.firstthings.com/article/2001/11/darwin-and-the-descent-of-morality).
113 DARWIN C. *The Descent of Man, and Selection in Relation to Sex*. New York: D. Appleton; 1872: Volume 1 p. 67.
114 *Ibid*. p. 69.
115 *Ibid*. p. 161-162.

to distance him from eugenics.[116]

But if conscience is merely an evolutionary construct which can be discarded as evolution progresses beyond a certain stage, one wonders what will take its place? What is to happen within a totalitarian regime? Must everybody then obey the dictates of the current ideology, since there is no natural moral law as a reference point for one's conscience? But if conscience may licitly be ignored, why did we expect the criminals from the Third Reich to have known better and therefore condemned them for their crimes? They thought they were following the evolutionary process, bringing the Aryan race to dominance, and only hastening what they thought would happen inevitably. Yet few accept that as an excuse.

The implicit, popular form of this Darwinian approach shies away from such extremes; its implication is that conscience allows society to grow harmoniously together, protecting the weaker and checking the stronger, and that this useful service will be possible one day without the help of conscience. However, this contradicts one of the key Darwinian laws of nature, which is the survival of the fittest with no regard for the weaker. Furthermore, what is supposed to take the place of conscience at a later stage of evolution? What else could hold people in check to this extent, making them disregard their own interests and desires for the sake of others? To believe in utilitarianism, the rational weighing of consequences and the realization that in the long run it will be best for everyone if we follow certain rules, as replacing the dictates of conscience, is to be hopelessly naïve. It fails to acknowledge human nature, which will – if not held back by some real absolutes – seek in most cases the immediate gratification of its own desires rather than serving the common good with its long-term good consequences. One would think that the 20th century and what we have seen so far of the 21st would be enough to disprove belief in this kind of progress. If there is an inbuilt mechanism in nature or history, which would warrant this, then it has failed to be validated so far.

Furthermore, one cannot speak of conscience as a survival mechanism, at least not for the individual, since often enough, it leads to situations where a person has to act against her own self-interest and even risk her life. Just like Socrates called himself the gadfly of Athenian society, so our conscience is our gadfly, continuously stirring us, warning us, raising our awareness towards things we would much rather not think about, prompting us to do things which are uncomfortable and even dangerous. If it is nothing but the inbuilt mechanism of society to protect itself, then the evolution from instinct to conscience seems to have been a poor adaptation, one that should have been eliminated by natural selection. In fact, Darwin was "largely stumped" in trying to explain the evolution of human conscience and very little work has been done on the evolution of conscience since his time.[117] The Darwinian

---

116 WIKE. *Darwin and the Descent...*, (accessed on 17.11.2014, at: http://www.firstthings.com/article/2001/11/darwin-and-the-descent-of-morality).

117 WASON P. Overview: *The Evolution of Conscience A Workshop of the John Templeton Foundation* (28 April-1 May 2010). Santa Fe; 2010 (accessed on 25.11.2014, at: http://symposia.templeton.org/evolution_of_conscience/index.html).

understanding of conscience is not a convincing theory and needs to be seen for what it is, namely a flawed hypothesis.

1.3.3 The Freudian Approach

Freud did much to shape the modern idea of conscience, as will become clear. Freud distinguishes between the id, the ego and the superego. Human beings are born with the id, which is basically the same as the instincts. The ego then develops in a physiological manner from the id under the influence of the external world. The superego, however, is formed through the parents' education, telling the child what it should and shouldn't do; culture, the social milieu, education and many other factors shape the superego as well, from which the moral conscience arises. Freud writes about the superego in *An Outline of Psychoanalysis* that it "continues to carry on the functions which have hitherto been performed by the people in the external world; it observes the ego, gives it orders, judges it, and threatens it with punishments, exactly like the parents whose place it has taken".[118] Hence, conscience is that within the superego which judges and threatens. Furthermore, conscience has a conscious and an unconscious part, which also guides our behavior. The superego, as Langston clarifies in his analysis on Freud, is similar to *synderesis*, as it was understood in the Middle Ages, namely as "repository of the agent's beliefs and dictates" while conscience applies these beliefs to specific cases and causes suffering, when it is not obeyed.[119]

A Freudian approach to conscience therefore sees in conscience the voice of the father, the voice of the superego, which needs to be overcome, since it shackles the person down and makes her feel bad about things she should really enjoy. However, only if her educators had a masochistic or puritanical worldview, would it make sense to shake off this view, but not conscience as such. For the individual is not determined by the way his conscience was shaped; he can eventually rise above it, by letting his conscience be formed by what is authentically right and true rather than warped. Going against the distorted morals of one's educators does not mean that one should discard conscience as such (though some do), but instead try to rectify one's conscience in light of the natural moral law. It is only in light of that law, that one can determine whether one's conscience has been distorted or not. This is the touchstone, which makes one able to judge the rightness of one's conscience.

That conscience is different from the superego becomes clear in cases where the person's conscience is opposed to that of her educators. Even people raised under totalitarian regimes can see through the lies and the injustice of the system on their own; their conscience tells them that they need to stand up against it, whatever the cost. Conscience is therefore something quite different and far above social constructs, Darwinian hypotheses, and psychological sicknesses. It is more than the superego or only "the psychological vestiges of childhood".[120]

---

118 Quoted in LANGSTON. *Conscience...*, p. 89.
119 *Ibid.* p. 91.
120 VISCHER. *Conscience and the Common Good...*, p. 64.

Education certainly has a big role to play in the formation of conscience, but it does not create it. Our conscience is an irreducible inner voice, which will speak up if it has not been completely squashed, despite the *Zeitgeist*, public opinion, social *milieu* and education.

Freud furthermore holds, according to Strohm, that guilt precedes the transgression rather than following upon it. Free-floating guilt causes dissatisfaction, which then finds some resolution in committing a crime.[121] However, one could interpret the phenomenon of free-floating guilt differently. Rather than guilt preceding the criminal act, one could persuasively argue that this guilt is either due to some former transgression, which the person hasn't repented; or it could be unfounded guilt, due to falsely inculcated beliefs. The right way to get rid of it would be to either address one's guilty past, repent and make reparation as far as this is possible, or to come to a full realization that the former belief-system was erroneous and that the guilty feelings are therefore unfounded. Either way offers an alternative to Freud's theory that guilt precedes rather than is subsequent to transgressions.

It is interesting to note, as Strohm points out, that despite his critique of conscience, Freud does not seem to think that we can do away with it. In "Mourning and Melancholia" he writes, "we shall count it, along with the censorship of consciousness and the testing of reality, among the great institutions of the ego".[122] It protects the common good by shackling the instincts of the individual, as he writes in "Civilization and its Discontents". He even suggests that society as a whole can develop a superego to further its interests. But how does he expect conscience to continue pursuing its vital role, when he deconstructs it and shows people that they are allowing themselves to be dominated by something oppressive and false? This is logically contradictory and psychologically unhealthy.

1.3.4 The Neurological Approach

Without going into details that would take us outside the confines of this dissertation's topic, I would like to criticize another variant of the above-mentioned theories, namely the neurological one.[123] It holds that conscience is simply a chemical reaction of our brain, something which happens despite us and for our greater good. Evolutionary biology rears again its ugly head here.

If conscience is only there for the purpose of one's own survival or that of one's species, it seems to be an example of flawed evolution. It demands sometimes that a whole people do things that could lead to their death. Why not stick to instinct, which would be much more reliable? Conscience seems a poor substitute, if we look at totalitarian regimes where the consciences of many are silenced or deformed. Again, the question arises, what the next evolutionary step

---

121 STROHM. *Conscience…*, p.68.
122 *Ibid.* p. 72.
123 BAHM AJ. *Theories of Conscience.* Ethics. 1965; 75 (2): 128-131, p. 131.

would be after the deconstruction of conscience. Mere reason, as I have noted earlier, seems a weak replacement and only utopians could think this would keep people in check.

The neurological interpretation of conscience is reductionist; it claims that conscience is "nothing but" brain-waves, neuro-transmitters etc. This presupposes that explanations need to refer to what is lower in order to understand something higher. In the same line of thought is the idea that love is "nothing but chemistry", justice "nothing but brain-waves" etc. But why would something lower necessarily explain something higher? This is a hypothesis, which requires some explanation in and of itself, for it is hard to fathom how something higher could arise out of something lower. Where does it get that extra lift, this new information, order, and purpose to bring out something so complex? Metaphysically speaking this is nonsense.

However, what about the fact that people with brain damage can lose their moral conscience and their capacity to empathize among other things? Does this not prove that conscience is simply a function of the brain? If the brain-chemistry is in order, then conscience will function; but if it isn't, then one has the case of a psychopath. But it does not follow from this necessarily that conscience is nothing but chemistry. Correct brainchemistry is only the condition for it to function well. In that case, a damaged brain would not meet the necessary conditions for conscience to raise its voice, just like a brain-injury might affect a person's capacity to think, see or hear.

Intuitively one tends to understand that doing evil is generally not simply the result of a chemical imbalance. That is why we distinguish in the exercise of the law between those who seem to have psychological issues, which might reduce their responsibility, and those who are "of sound mind" and should know better. We send the first into mental institutions, while we imprison the others.

1.4 Dealing with Objections

The conscientious objection debate has much to do with divergent understandings of conscience. How can one come to an understanding and consensus regarding conscientious objection if one operates with different concepts of conscience?[124] As I have shown so far, the main modern arguments against a recognition of conscience as a moral cognitive tool are based on moral relativism. I have attempted to disprove these and show the contradictory nature of moral relativism. If conscience is nothing but a construct, whatever its origin, then there is no compelling reason to make a special space for it within society. Some, of course, might still argue that it is valuable as a construct and should therefore not be casually discarded by society in general and the medical profession in particular. But it has still lost its justification and metaphysical foundation, and thus the most powerful reason for honoring it.

---

124 LAWRENCE, CURLIN. *Clash of Definitions…*, p. 10.

Another reason often tendered against respecting conscience within health-care is that it is a religious concept. Marcus Adam asserts, for example, that "religious conscience, regardless of the religion from which it develops, has no place in medical decisionmaking". [125] This fails to take into consideration that conscience is an anthropological reality, which is recognized by atheists and believers alike. Though its understanding became highly developed within a Christian context, it is by no means reducible to it (its roots in ancient Greece and Rome show this). The individual arguing that he cannot in good conscience perform a certain act does so because, to his mind, it contradicts morality, the dignity of the human person and because he does not want to incur moral guilt by doing it. We expect doctors in situations like those prevalent during the Third Reich to stand up against immoral orders and procedures, whether they are religiously minded or not.

The fact that society is pluralistic and that many operate with a highly individualistic understanding of conscience does make the debate more difficult. This is a different question altogether, however, from saying that conscience is therefore totally subjective. One can argue rationally and convincingly for an anthropologically founded understanding of conscience that escapes the merely subjective or ideological winds by letting itself be formed by the natural moral law and a wider ethical community, even if many do not agree with it. Conscience's metaphysical foundation is a different question from how one can communicate convincingly with people who have a different understanding of it. Can one argue that a person should follow her conscience, even if it is nothing but a whim or the projection of one's superego? My claim is that one can, though the argument is much stronger when it is based on an objective understanding of conscience; the consequences of incurring moral guilt by thinking one is committing serious moral evil, even if one is *de facto* not doing anything bad, are so serious that the person needs to have this freedom vouchsafed. [126]

1.5. What is the importance of conscience?

In agreement with the view that it is a primary right of the first importance not to have one's conscience violated, the great human rights instruments of modern international law recognize this right. The 1948 Universal Declaration of Human Rights speaks of conscience in the preamble, article 1 and article 18 where it says: "Everyone has the right to freedom of

---

125 ADAMS MP. *Conscience and Conflict*. Am J Bioeth. 2007; 7 (12): 28-29, p. 29.
126 Hogan speaks about two meanings of conscience that are used at the same time within the Catholic tradition and which are in conflict in the documents of Vatican II. She thinks they are used without distinction and cause confusion. For example, in *Gaudium et Spes*, as Hogan points out, conscience is first used as obedience to an objective moral law, and then later in the quote as the voice of God echoing in one's depths, regardless of whether one is a Christian or not. Hogan fails to understand that God's voice and the moral law are the same, and that there is only a conflict when conscience is erroneous. HOGAN. *Confronting the Truth...*, p. 111; PAUL VI. Gaudium et Spes..., §16.

thought, conscience and religion".[127] Article 9 of the 1950 Convention for the Protection of Human Rights and Fundamental Freedoms and even the 2004 draft European Constitution in article II-70 dedicated to fundamental rights, recognize freedom of conscience. Article 18 of the 1966 International Covenant on Civil and Political Rights states unequivocally that, "everyone shall have the right to freedom of thought, conscience and religion".[128]

I will argue in my thesis that moral conscience should be formed by the natural law, which it implicitly refers to. However, even though moral relativists will miss some essential aspects of why going against one's conscience is an unmitigated moral evil, they can still grasp part of the issue. A person going against her moral conscience will have to live with a "split self" and in a schizophrenic way. If she goes against a belief she holds to be right and true, she thereby undermines her own integrity. How can she live with herself afterwards? She will probably have a bad conscience, sensing deep down that she should not have committed this evil. She might try to argue herself out of this situation, saying that she was, after all, not free, that it doesn't really matter, that she will try to make up for this etc. But nothing can undo the fact that she contradicted herself in an important and fundamental way. In consequence, she might deaden her conscience and even become morally blind, generally speaking. At the very least, it is clear that she will have lost something: her integrity, her peace of mind, her good conscience. An inner contradiction will have entered into her center.

This, for Hannah Arendt, is at the bottom of her concept of "thoughtfulness": the person is in dialogue with herself when having to make a moral choice; if she thinks matters through, she will not choose something, which undermines herself and her basic principles. In her article "Thinking and Moral Considerations", she contrasts Socrates with Eichmann. The former sought to know himself and conversed with himself while the latter did not engage in much self-reflection.[129] One could rightly argue that this enlightenment approach does away with the force and drama of the moral choice, watering it down to nothing more than a rational decision. But at least it shows that somebody like Arendt who does not want to refer to an objective moral law can still be strongly opposed to going against one's moral conscience. She saw that there is something within the human person, her very structure, which is harmed by doing so. It is furthermore true that disregard for the importance and value of conscience puts citizens at the mercy of any ideology and totalitarian regime. For what will keep them from submitting to tremendous ideological pressures if they have already undermined and silenced their consciences?

127 UNITED NATIONS GENERAL ASSEMBLY. *Universal Declaration of Human Rights*. (10 December 1948). Paris; 1948 (accessed on 19.09.2014, at: http://www.un.org/en/documents/udhr/index.shtml#a18).
128 Id. *International Covenant on Civil and Political Rights*. (23 March 1976). New York; 1976 (accessed on 19.09.2014, at: http://www.ohchr.org/EN/ProfessionalInterest/Pages/CCPR.aspx).
129 ARENDT H. *Thinking and Moral Considerations: A Lecture*. Social Research. 1971; 38 (3): 417-446.

In *L'Enracinement*, Simone Weil speaks of something sacred which is at the center of every human person. This is due to her capacity to relate to a reality not of this world, namely the absolute good. To try to destroy this capacity or impinge this orientation in the person is a terrible crime in her eyes, since the good is the finality of every human being. It hits him in his core, if I make it difficult or impossible for him to reach it. Forcing somebody to do evil would amount to a kind of sacrilege.[130]

Sometimes human beings are confronted with seemingly conflicting obligations. In totalitarian regimes, these instances become frequent. They put the person in a situation of having to choose between obeying a positive law (like discriminating against the Jews) and their own life. The stark alternatives are therefore heroism or moral corruption. This should not be so, and Weil therefore sees the urgent need for a constitution and government, which would seek to avoid such clashes arising at all. Protecting the right to conscientious objection, I would argue, is an essential protection for the rights of the human person. They have to do with her core, her orientation, and her finality.

Doing evil or good has a tremendous impact on the human person who undermines or fulfills her potential by doing the one or the other. Hence, we grasp that the human person determines through her choices, through her acts and omissions, what kind of person she becomes. In the first case, there is a transcendence, a growing beyond her self-interest that comes about by responding to the good; in the latter case, the person becomes increasingly locked up in herself, in her own desires and ideological fiction. One could speak of an implosion of the person in the latter case, of her becoming simply a shell of herself. By failing to respond to moral absolutes, by neglecting to recognize that human beings are transcendent beings meant to respond to the good, they become caricatures of themselves. They become subject to the whim of their desires and of the current *Zeitgeist*, and have lost their moral backbone. With their moral conscience, they have also lost their hearts. For they are no longer able to feel for others who, according to their ideology, are "unworthy of life" (*lebensunwertes Leben*).[131] Hence, Eichmann could feel revolt at the blood spilled in the execution of Jews in the Holocaust, but not experience any sympathy for their suffering nor come to the conclusion that exterminating the Jews was morally wrong.[132]

---

130 WEIL S. *Oeuvres complètes* V, 2: Écrits de New York et de Londres (1943). Paris: Gallimard; 2013: p.97-99.

131 In the Third Reich, the doctors became involved in the extermination programs often out of fear and cowardice, especially fear of punishment or of being ostracized. "Whatever proportions these crimes finally assumed, it became evident to all who investigated them that they had started from small beginnings. The beginnings at first were only a subtle shift in emphasis in the basic attitude of the physicians. It started with the acceptance of the attitude, basic in the euthanasia movement, that there is such a thing as life not worthy to be lived". ALEXANDER L. *Medical Science under Dictatorship*. N Engl J Med. 1949; 241 (2): 39-47, p. 44.

132 ARENDT H. *Eichmann in Jerusalem: A Report on the Banality of Evil*. New York: Penguin Books; 2006: p. 88-89.

In her article, "Newman on Conscience and our Culture", Teresa Iglesias Rozas shows that Newman understood conscience "to preserve and fulfill our moral identity and integrity".[133] It is our inbuilt way of protecting our inner core, that which defines us, in not letting us get away with what contradicts our moral principles. This confirms its essential role and that the State does well to respect it.

Conscience, as I have tried to show, is key to understanding the human person. As a moral agent, she needs conscience as her personal moral compass in order to navigate around the continuous challenges and moral questions she has to address every day. Trying to explain conscience away, leaves us with a fundamental human experience unexplained. The attempts to replace it with something else are unsatisfactory and are more hypothetical and speculative than assuming conscience itself exists; for it is a familiar reality to almost every person. When society fails to acknowledge its existence and does not provide protections for individuals to follow their consciences, this fosters grave conflicts. Either the persons in question will heroically obey their conscience, whatever the cost, or they will lose their moral integrity with all the devastating effects that flow from this on society at large. Everybody needs conscience as his personal gadfly, just like Athens needed Socrates as its voice of conscience. Lynn Wardle points out how James Madison and Thomas Jefferson viewed conscience rights as foundational: "If you demand that a man betray his conscience, you have eliminated the only moral basis for his fidelity to the rule of law, and have destroyed the moral foundation for democracy. Thus, protection of rights of conscience is necessary for the rule of law in a republican form of government".[134]

This chapter has set the stage to investigate the rights of conscience of medical professionals. Since they have positions of great responsibility and power in a field where moral probity is essential, their consciences should be particularly well developed and protected. Otherwise, we run the serious risk of health care personnel arrogating to themselves the right to become masters over life and death or allowing others to do so in the high stress and frequently conflictual situations of hospital or medical decisionmaking. Medical professionals are already under tremendous pressure to submit to the demands of patients, medical administrators and government regulations and laws. Undermining the right and responsibility of doctors and other health professionals to exercise their consciences in their medical practice is akin to society shooting itself in the foot. This, however, will be shown more clearly in the following chapters.

---

133 ROZAS. *Newman on Conscience…*, p. 39.
134 WARDLE LD. *Protection of Health-Care Providers' Rights of Conscience in American Law: Present, Past, and Future.* Ave Maria Law Rev. 2010. 9 (1): 1-46, p. 8.

CHAPTER 2:

HUMAN RIGHTS AND CONSCIENCE

The modern human rights regime is a source of pride for the West, yet has proven problematic in recent decades.[135] Bolstering human rights with a philosophical foundation that can be accepted as widely as the rights themselves and providing acceptable boundaries to the concept has been difficult. In consequence, defending and enforcing these rights over and against nations who disregard them in the name of cultural diversity and national sovereignty is not an easy task. A proliferation of "new rights", some of which easily conflict with previously recognized rights, compounds the problems. I will try to offer a metaphysical and personalist foundation for human rights, which, if accepted, would be a solid bulwark against abuses originating from confusion and relativism. However, even if the problems surrounding human rights cannot be easily resolved, I will also argue that even within a context where human rights are thought to be lacking a metaphysical foundation, one can still argue rationally for the acceptance of conscientious objection as a human right. For the right to conscience is well established in human rights declarations and treaties, and its rejection leads to grave crises and wounds within the human person.

2.1 A Historical Overview of the Question of Human Rights

Human rights as a matter of international legal protection have made great strides in the modern era even though the idea can be traced very far back in time.[136] Important precedents from ancient history include the rights of citizens of Greek city-states and the Stoic philosophers from the Hellenistic period who believed that natural rights were held by all men, regardless of citizenship, simply because of their humanity.[137] The French Declaration of the Rights of Man and of the Citizen from 1789 and the Bill of Rights added to the US Constitution in 1791 are two milestones from the 18th century on the way to the explosion of international human rights declarations and treaties following the Second World War and continuing into the 21st century. A core insight concerning modern human rights is that they are meant to be universal legal rights and not just moral claims.[138] Some say that 1945, with the adoption of the United Nations (UN) Charter, marked the advent of the protection

---

135 DONNELLY J. *International Human Rights: A Regime Analysis*. Int Organ. 1986; 40 (3): 599-642, p. 616. (accessed on 28.11.2014, at: http://ernie.itpir.wm.edu/pdf/NewArticles/Liberal/2706821.pdf).

136 PERRY MJ. *The Idea of Human Rights: Four Inquiries*. Oxford: Oxford University Press; 2000: p. 5.

137 CRANSTON M. *What are Human Rights?* London: The Bodley Head Ltd; 1973: p. 2.

138 HOOKER B. *On Human Rights* [Book Review]. Oxf J Leg Stud. 2010; 30 (1): 193-205.

of human rights entering international law in a systematic way.[139] In article 55 of the charter it states that the UN will promote; "universal respect for, and observance of, human rights and fundamental freedoms for all without distinction as to race, sex, language, or religion".[140] Following the crimes against humanity committed before and during World War II and the Nuremberg War Crimes Trials, a consensus developed that human rights must be proclaimed and defended internationally. Composing and proclaiming the Universal Declaration of Human Rights (UDHR) in 1948 was and remains one of the most celebrated acts of the United Nations. The Soviet Union (USSR) nevertheless successfully blocked the UDHR from being a binding treaty document by their insistence that they would only support a manifesto.[141] The enumeration of rights in that declaration was the fruit of much debate, and, as mentioned in chapter one, conscience is found in the preamble, articles 1 and 18.[142] The end result of the UDHR was nevertheless only a proclamation of principles without the juridical force of an international treaty. Despite this inauspicious beginning, some now consider that the UDHR has become part of customary international law.[143]

Work began almost immediately to craft international human rights treaties. The International Covenant on Civil and Political Rights (ICCPR) was adopted in 1966 and came into force in 1976. At the same time, the separate International Covenant on Economic, Social and Cultural Rights (ICESCR) was adopted and also came into force in 1976. The UN convened the first global conference on human rights in Teheran, Iran in 1968 to commemorate the twentieth anniversary of the Universal Declaration of Human Rights. Decolonization and Cold War concerns dominated this world conference as is evident from the final Proclamation of Teheran outcome document.[144]

During the Cold War, the USSR and Communist Block led a coalition of nations urging the equality of economic, cultural and social rights as opposed to the traditional primacy of civil and political rights.[145] Since communist states were notorious for their denial of basic civil and political liberties, they tried to shift attention to other rights where they claimed higher levels of success, i.e. equality of economic participation, access to cultural events, etc. With the end of the Cold War following the collapse of the USSR and its European client states, the deadlock over civil and political rights vs. economic, cultural and social rights was ironically broken by the UN's adoption of a position most closely resembling the one

---

139 DAVIDSON S. *Human Rights*. Buckingham: Open University Press; 1993: p. 1.
140 UNITED NATIONS GENERAL ASSEMBLY. *Charter of the United Nations* (26 June 1945). San Francisco; 1945: Art. 55. (accessed on 09.10.2014 at: https://www.un.org/en/documents/charter/chapter9.shtml).
141 CRANSTON. *What are Human Rights?...*, p. 53.
142 UNITED NATIONS GENERAL ASSEMBLY. *Universal Declaration...*, Preamble, Art. 1, Art. 18.
143 DONNELLY. *International Human Rights...*, p. 608.
144 INTERNATIONAL CONFERENCE ON HUMAN RIGHTS. *Proclamation of Teheran* (13 May 1968). Teheran; 1968 (accessed on 09.28.2014, at: http://www1.umn.edu/humanrts/instree/l2ptichr.htm).
145 SHELTON. *Hierarchy of Norms...*, p. 302.

formerly championed by the communists. The most likely reason for this was the adoption of a similarly critical stance towards the predominance of civil and political rights by the governments of many developing nations.[146]

In 1993, the UN convened the Vienna World Conference on Human Rights, and its outcome document, The Vienna Declaration and Programme of Action (VDPA),[147] was perceived as going counter to the Cold War era qualitative distinction generally supported by Western democratic governments, ranking civil and political rights above economic, cultural and social rights. Former UN High Commissioner for Human Rights, Navi Pillay, reflected on the 20th anniversary of the Vienna Conference that, "many of us were very concerned about the risk that the Conference would break apart with many countries favouring the primacy, or exclusivity, of civil and political rights; and others [were] arguing for the primacy of economic, social and cultural rights."[148] The Vienna conference created the position of United Nations High Commissioner for Human Rights and the Office of the United Nations High Commissioner for Human Rights (OHCHR).

Strangely, in the midst of all these controversies the difficulty of grounding human rights was rarely addressed. What foundation would be solid enough to withstand the assaults of new ideologies? Thinkers over the years have posited different ways of justifying human rights philosophically, for example through their positive results, founding them on consensus, on a social contract, or on the human will. I will briefly look at the difficulties surrounding a definition of human rights and critique some of these positions before attempting to show the truth, rationality and advantages of a metaphysical and personalist foundation of human rights.

2.2 Human Rights

Basic human rights are generally considered to be universal; it is in a way the whole point of coming up with a theory of human rights that they are applicable to everybody. Human beings possess them independently of their ethnicity, social background, convictions, talents or lack thereof. They have human rights by virtue of being human.But what does one exactly mean by "rights"? Its legal and philosophical meanings are manifold. In his article,

---

145 SHELTON. *Hierarchy of Norms...*, p. 302.

146 TAYLOR PE *From Environmental to Ecological Human Rights: A New Dynamic in International Law?*. Georget Int Environ Law Rev. 10 (1997): 309-397, p. 320.

147 WORLD CONFERENCE ON HUMAN RIGHTS. *Vienna Declaration and Programme of Action* (25 June 1993). Vienna; 1993 (accessed on 21.11.2014, at: http://www.ohchr.org/Documents/ ProfessionalInterest/ vienna.pdf).

148 UNITED NATIONS HUMAN RIGHTS OFFICE OF THE HIGH COMMISSIONER. Vienna *Declaration and Programme of Action: 20 Years Working for Your Rights*: 1993 World Conference on Human Rights. New York: OHCR and the Department of Public Information. 2013 (accessed on 21.11.2014, at: http://www. ohchr.org/Documents/ Events/OHCHR20/VDPAbooklet English.pdf).

"The Philosophic Foundations of Human Rights", Jerome Shestack points out some of these, delineating the difficulties of those grappling with this notion. Having a right could mean that one is entitled to something, or it could refer to an immunity or then again to a privilege. When calling rights inalienable, does this mean that there are no limits tied to them? Or that human rights have priority, with those wishing to limit them having to make a weighty case before they are overturned? Or does inalienable mean that a right must be respected except if another moral principle allows for its curtailment?[149]

If one thinks of a right as a claim against a government to desist from certain acts like torture or murder, then this is quite different from seeing in it a privilege that is granted by the State and which can therefore be curtailed. Furthermore, if rights are considered to be claims and include, for example, the right to free education and paid vacations, does this mean the State is obliged in all circumstances to meet them? Or are they more goals that one aspires to, knowing full well that reality will always fall short of meeting them?[150]

Though he points out many possible meanings of rights, Shestack fails to give any guidance as how best to define human rights. He does not distinguish, for example, between different kinds of rights and their hierarchical order of importance (something I will argue for in the second half of this chapter), thereby confusing matters more. Thomas D. Williams in his book, Who is My Neighbor?, gives a phenomenological and linguistic analysis to clarify the term. He shows that there are four components of rights, namely "the possessor of the right, the possessor of the duty to respect or satisfy the right, the thing or action in question, and a reciprocal moral relationship that binds them all together".[151] A right is always something one has; the owner possesses the right, whether he exercises it or not. One always speaks about a right to something; merely speaking about a right without reference to what one has as right, does not make any sense. Thomas D. Williams thinks of human rights as a moral right or faculty. [152] He also points out that the term "right" connotes moral justice; the implication and whole point of rights is justly to claim a certain right, asking others to respond to it. Human rights are furthermore other-directed; they address themselves to another to perform a duty vis-à-vis one's right.

In his article, "Philosophische Grundlagen der Menschenrechte", Josef Seifert clarifies the meaning of human rights. A right is a claim of one person to another; if a contract has been entered into, then this claim is addressed to a specific person. If a fundamental natural right like the right to life is at stake, then it is an absolute claim not to be killed that is addressed to everybody.[153] Though they overlap, human rights are different from moral obligations. The

149 SHESTACK JJ. *The Philosophical Foundations of Human Rights*. Hum Rts Q. 20 (1998): 201-234, p. 203.
150 *Ibid*. p. 204.
151 WILLIAMS TD. *Who Is My Neighbor? Personalism and the Foundations of Human Rights*.
Washington DC: Catholic University of America Press; 2005: p. 8-9.
152 WILLIAMS. *Who Is My Neighbor?...*, p. 5-6.
153 SEIFERT J. *Philosophische Grundlagen der Menschenrechte: Zur Verteidigung des Menschen*. Prima Philosophia. 1988; 5 (4): 339-370, p. 344.

latter require much more from the agent, for example the right intention, inner attitudes and value-responses, which human rights do not demand. As long as one respects the right to life of the other, even if one wishes him dead, one has respected his human right. The State generally only prosecutes human rights violations (when they are reflected in the constitution and/or legislation) and not transgressions that lie only in the ethical realm.

Human rights, as Seifert explains, are not so much "human" in that they are different from rights regarding animals or non-living objects (and one cannot speak of "rights" in those cases). Instead, they are human because they are based on the nature of the human person rather than on positive laws (though they are meant to be reflected in the latter). Secondly, they are called human rights because they are central to man's humanity, to his destiny and happiness.[154] After having critiqued various theories contradicting this metaphysical grounding of human rights, I will attempt to show the validity of this claim in greater depth.

Human rights claim a certain objectivity. Otherwise, they would be at the arbitrary mercy of a tyrant. One therefore refers to them often in situations where the state does not recognize them, thereby pointing to a reality over which the state has no legitimate power.[155] Their existence does not depend on people's perception, recognition or liking. Basic human rights are inborn and not acquired. They are inalienable, i.e. they cannot be undone by myself or someone else or the State. They are also "untouchable". They are addressed to others, and not to myself (I can act in ways that contradict my human dignity, but I cannot go against my own human rights). They are universal in that they are grounded on unchangeable human nature, as I will show, and are in that sense neither historically nor culturally relative (though they have been discovered and articulated within specific cultures at particular points in time).

2.2.1 A Critique of Various Human Rights Foundations
2.2.1.1 Interest Theory: A Utilitarian Definition of Human Rights[156]

Utilitarianism proclaims that there is no such thing as justice or the good as such. The ultimate measuring rod for everything is usefulness. When we say that something is good or just, what we really mean, according to this theory, is that it is useful to us in some way or to society at large (and therefore to us indirectly). This reductionist theory lends itself also to a justification of human rights. For prudential reasons, it is in the interests of everybody that human rights be recognized, since it means one's own shall also be respected. Hence, human

---

154 *Ibid.* p. 345.
155 *Ibid.* p. 345-346.
156 Underlying a utilitarian definition of human rights as well as consensus theory is positivism. It denies any foundations to human rights other than those declared by the state, and can be critiqued in a similar way as these other two theories. SHESTACK. The Philosophical Foundations..., p. 208-9.

rights are ultimately based on self-interest.[157] Though an individual might not just now be in a category of people who are in danger of being eliminated, he might one day (if he becomes old, handicapped or loses his mind etc.). Hence, for the protection of all and for the greater good of society, which cannot function well nor have happy citizens in an atmosphere where nobody is safe, human rights are useful tools.

The beauty of this theory is that it is satisfactory to the vast majority of people and appeals to commonality. It does not depend on any profound philosophical or metaphysical considerations, does not require the acceptance of a natural law, and is acceptable to the relativist as well as to the secular mind. Because of its universal appeal, it seems that this understanding of human rights would be very fruitful. John Finnis is a good representative of interest-theory, a variant of utilitarianism, since in his book, Natural Law and Natural Rights, he bases his foundation of human rights on the interest of individuals in a stable society. He justifies human rights in their capacity to assure the necessary conditions for well-being. He lists seven "basic forms of human good" which need to be respected for the flourishing of the human person, namely life, the acquisition of knowledge as an end in and of itself, play, aesthetic experience, sociability and friendship, practical reasonableness, and finally religion.[158]

However, there are a number of problems with this theory. If usefulness is the ultimate value, what happens if it turns out that human rights are no longer useful? A regime similar to the Third Reich or the Soviet Union might say that the most useful way of furthering the advent of the master race or the victory of the proletariat, is that only the useful and fit should live. In the name of this useful goal, the human rights of some citizens will therefore be abolished. Since there is nothing else to appeal to like the injustice of such a proceeding, usefulness having become the ultimate end, one has no leg to stand on. Human rights have become simply a facet of a group's self-interest. One could, of course, argue that human rights based on self-interest would not allow for such a regime as the Third Reich or the USSR to arise, at least if people thought sufficiently about their self-interest. For even the powerful are in danger of being eliminated at some point, as the Roehm-putsch or the show-trials under Stalin proved, and would do well therefore to think of society as a whole. But this assumes that people always have primarily their own self-interest at heart and that this is the strongest motivation to act reasonably. Experience has shown, however, that people may well be willing to sacrifice themselves for the sake of a cause though it goes against their self-interest. Furthermore, the powerful fool themselves into thinking that they are invulnerable and have no interest in promoting human rights. One could object, however, that nothing will prevent those who are willing to walk over other people from doing so; a metaphysical foundation for human rights

---

157 NICKEL J. *Making Sense of Human Rights: Philosophical Reflections on the Universal Declaration of Human Rights*. Berkeley: University of California Press; 1987: p. 84; FAGAN A. *Human Rights*. Internet Encyclopedia of Philosophy, 1987. (accessed on 20.11.2014, at: http://www.iep.utm.edu/hum-rts).
158 FINNIS J. *Natural Law and Natural Rights*. Oxford: Clarendon Press; 2011. p. 86-90.

will prevent them just as much or as little as one based on self-interest. This is plausible, of course. But the appeal to what is morally right nevertheless has more leverage than pleas to safeguard self-interest, as I will show later.

Furthermore, utilitarian theory makes the anthropological assumption that human beings' first and foremost motivation is self-interest. When Maximilian Kolbe volunteered to give his life for another condemned concentration camp inmate, he was obviously not motivated by self-interest. To reduce everything to self-interest ultimately means seeing human beings as incapable of transcending themselves. This does not do justice to heroes, saints and some great artists, for example, who deny themselves the fulfillment of their own needs for the sake of others or their work.

Another problem with this theory is that it presupposes, as some have pointed out, that the minimal conditions for a decent life are not culturally relative. Some cultures, particularly in Asia, see rights as less important than virtues.[159] Furthermore, it implies that all people are equally vulnerable. In reality, living conditions are very unequal, and a poor person in the poorest part of the world is much more in danger of having her basic human rights violated than a wealthy person in a "first world" country. Why should the latter feel compelled to help the former, since it does not seem to affect her own selfinterest in any way? It seems much more reasonable in a way to presuppose that those people who donate money for people in need on the other side of the globe or who stand up for their human rights do it out of the goodness of their hearts, because they feel pity for those suffering and recognize their fundamental human dignity.

Once one introduces usefulness into human affairs as the supreme criterion, everything deteriorates and becomes inhumane very quickly. When it is introduced into health care and bioethics, there is soon no compelling reason to care for those who have little or no chance of improvement. The Nazis called this lebensunwertes Leben (life unworthy of life), and we know where this kind of thinking led. The negative practical consequences of utilitarianism pushed to an extreme in certain historical cases have shown its flaws as being frankly horrible.[160]

A utilitarian theory can only work in society if people are willing to look at the good of society as a whole rather than their immediate self-interest. However, the vague promise that something will eventually benefit me tends to be much less persuasive than immediate gratification. Utilitarianism therefore only provides a very weak protection for those who cannot defend themselves. It has the further disadvantage of making the rationalization of immoral actions on a vast scale by unscrupulous persons holding the reigns of power quite easy.

---

159 SEN A. *Development as Freedom. Oxford*: Oxford University Press; 1999: p. 228.
160 A utilitarian ethics permeated Nazism and Marxism.

2.2.1.2 Consensus Theory

Consensus theory is another reductionist approach, for it denies the existence of objective truth and morality. Instead, everything that is called "true" or "right" can be explained and justified by consensus. It seems a fair and democratic procedure, for it makes everything depend on the majority rather than appealing to a truth others may not see or acknowledge. Human rights according to consensus theory are therefore considered universal in the sense that they are, as Jack Donnelly puts it, "almost universally accepted – at least in word, or as ideal standards".[161] This approach avoids the complications of agreeing on a common anthropology. According to Donnelly, most cultures have gone beyond moralities that distinguish between insiders and outsiders, and moral relativism notwithstanding, the widespread consensus on human rights is in consequence a sufficient basis from which to operate.

As Freeman points out in his article, "The Philosophical Foundations of Human Rights", Donnelly "moves from consensus to moral obligation on the communitarian ground that the moral beliefs of large majorities are binding on dissenting minorities".[162] Yet, as Donnelly himself would agree, majorities can very well be wrong, as the difficulties surrounding the abolition of slavery showed. Even if everybody, the victims included, were to agree that they have no human rights, this would not make slavery anymore right or justifiable. Hence, consensus can never be the basis for human rights, though it is true that the wider the consensus is the higher chances are that they will be respected.

The very fact that one needs to appeal to human rights usually means that they have been denied at least on a practical level. If consensus is what they depend upon for their validity, then they have a very weak foundation.[163] However, it is essential that a rational foundation for human rights be sought, otherwise they are at the absolute mercy of passions and ideologies. Some philosophers such as Rorty have claimed that it is pointless to seek such a philosophical foundation, but their position has been proven wrong by the many human rights abuses done in the name of the sovereignty of the State or of cultural relativism.[164] If mere custom or prejudice is the basis for human rights, then what determines which customs and prejudices are right and which are wrong? There has to be an external criterion against which one can judge them. The foundations of human rights need to have some universality and objectivity to be valid. Rorty denies such an objective measuring-rod; his idea of truth is that it is relative to somebody's perspective without there being a super-perspective by which one could judge diverse opinions.[165]

---

161 Quoted by FREEMAN M. *The Philosophical Foundations of Human Rights*. Hum Rights Q. 1994; 16: 491-514, p. 491; DONNELLY J. *Universal Human Rights in Theory and Practice*. Ithaca: Cornell University Press; 1989: p. 1, 23-27, 112-114.
162 *Ibid*. p. 492.
163 *Ibid*. p. 492-493.
164 *Ibid*. p. 495.
165 RORTY R. *Contingency, Irony and Solidarity*. Cambridge: Cambridge University Press; 1989: p. 63, 27.

Yet human beings have a strong inner sense about what is right and wrong, when they themselves have been violated in some way. Dworkin in his defense of natural rights (natural in the sense that they are not based on contracts, conventions or legislation) proposes two ways of explaining this inner sense. The one is that human rights are inherent to human beings and can be discovered intuitively, which is the position I defend. The other one is a "constructive" model, holding that basic principles have been worked into a coherent program of action over time, which is Dworkin's position.[166] The problem with Dworkin's theory is the same as that of other cultural relativists. There is no solid, rational foundation for weighing one theory against another, for preferring one over another, except for pragmatic considerations (a theory I criticized in the previous point) or conventions. So the basis for Dworkin's natural rights is precisely the one he is critical of in his opponents, namely contracts and conventions. He has no leg to stand on. Furthermore, as Freeman points out, the cultural relativism of these human rights defenders is the same as that of human rights' opponents. By using it as a pragmatic basis for human rights theories, they are playing into the hands of those who want to abolish human rights both on a theoretical as well as on a pragmatic level. What is needed is, in reality, a meta-ethical foundation, as Freeman calls it, or, as I would say, a metaphysical one.[167]

2.2.1.3 Will-Theory

Will theorists hold that human rights are philosophically founded on man's capacity for freedom. Freedom is what is distinctive about human action and should therefore be at the core of the defense of human rights.[168] H.L.A. Hart, for example, defends the idea that all rights are reducible to the right to be free, which Henry Shue extends to include the safety from violence and the necessary conditions for survival. Alan Gewirth argues that human rights are founded on human beings' capacity to act rationally and purposefully. The two preconditions for being able to act freely and with purpose are freedom and well-being, and therefore every individual is entitled to them. This, however, means accepting other people's claims to the same fundamental rights, and Gewirth calls this the "principle of generic consistency". He argues that there is therefore a fundamental right to life that is absolute and cannot be overridden for any reason.[169]

Gewirth holds that human rights are based on necessary truths, and are therefore not at the mercy of cultural change (though a culture may well deny certain rights, while promoting others). These truths are based on the nature of moral precepts that are always addressed

---

166 DWORKIN R. *Taking Rights Seriously*. London: Bloomsbury Academic; 2013: p. 197-200.
167 FREEMAN. *Philosophical Foundations…*, p. 501.
168 FAGAN *Human Rights…*(accessed on 20.11.2014, at: http://www.iep.utm.edu/hum-rts)
169 *Ibid.*

to a person who can choose and can act accordingly. The generic features of action, namely freedom and intentionality, provide the necessary content to morality.[170] Agents generally act in view of something they perceive as being good, at least for them, and must therefore view their freedom as good. They must therefore perceive as good also the conditions for the exercise for this freedom ranging from life to health. The implication, according to Gewirth, is that as an agent every human being must requirem certain rights to be able to act freely. It is so because, as Freeman summarizes Gewirth, "a claim to one's rights is implicit in agency itself".[171] The rights to freedom and wellbeing are moral and human rights, for they demand recognition by every agent regarding other agents, whether they are actual or only potential agents.[172] Human rights regard those goods that are necessary for the possibility of successful action; they do not depend on the kinds of choices made. Therefore, "agency is both a metaphysical and a moral basis for human dignity", as Freeman summarizes Gewirth, and is the basis of human rights.

A significant problem with this theory is that it depends on a human being's capacity to act autonomously, which might be curtailed or completely obstructed by dementia, coma, or mental diseases. Would people with these conditions not possess any human rights? Stretched further, it would mean that anybody sleeping would lose his human rights during sleep. One can, of course, circumvent this problem – which Gewirth does - by pointing out that every human being prospectively or potentially has the capacity to act autonomously, but this does not seem enough; for if our belief borders on certainty that somebody may never (again) possess this capacity, then this person would lose her human rights. A way out of this is to argue that human rights are based on human dignity, which is unalterable. However, Gewirth rejects this approach, calling it tautological, since it presupposes what it seeks to prove. Furthermore, the concept of human dignity is abstract and its meaning contestable, he claims.[173]

2.2.1.4 Social-Contract Theory

The theory of the social contract is based on the idea that human beings were originally in a state of nature, but then entered into a social contract to form a body politic. In Thomas Hobbes' view, the original state of humanity was defined by continuous wars against

---

170 GEWIRTH, A. *Reason and Morality*. Chicago: University of Chicago Press; 1981. p. 27.

171 FREEMAN. *Philosophical Foundations...*, p. 506.

172 *Ibid*. p. 507.

173 Ibid. These arguments are flawed. As I will show later on, basic data or "last things" cannot be proven by anything beyond them. However, one can make a philosophical analysis of then, delineating their essential features, and distinguishing them from things with which they might easily be confused. This is anything but tautological. Furthermore, that something is abstract or contestable is a purely utilitarian evaluation and says nothing about the truth or falsity of something. Everything is contestable, for that matter, Gewirth's theory included.

each other, and people feared for their lives and possessions. The social contract was the only way of protecting life and limb and creating a peaceful society. John Locke, however, posited an original state of humanity characterized by freedom and equality. Jean-Jacques Rousseau believed the social contract's primary virtue was to defend collectively liberty and order, and to do justice, thereby instituting a morality people in the state of nature were lacking.[174]

There are a fair number of problems with this theory. Since interest-theory also presupposes an implicit social contract, the arguments raised against interest-theory can be levelled against this approach as well. Further objections raised against it would be that it is unclear how and when this contract is or has been entered into and by whom. What exactly is its content and can it change? How are the rights of minorities recognized, if their content is determined by the majority? If it is in the interest of all that the rights of minorities should also recognized, then the same arguments levelled against interest-theory can be used here as well (for example, the powerful preferring their own interests to that of the majority).

2.3 Metaphysical Grounding of Human Rights: A Personalist Perspective

To some it may seem that seeking a metaphysical foundation for human rights is a futile experiment. Aladsair MacIntyre thinks human rights are pure figments of the imagination like witches and unicorns. Trying to argue for them is about as futile as rationally supporting the latter.[175] Some think it is dogmatic and therefore unphilosophical to do so, for it means pointing to a reality in its own right which cannot be disproved. But what else than metaphysics, i.e. referring to the very nature of the human person could give us a similarly solid foundation for human rights? That there is much disagreement about aposition does not mean that it is not rational, but could simply indicate that human beings are easily swayed by public opinion and personal interest from recognizing the truth. Rational inquiry, when dealing with "last things" that are sui generis, means making a close analysis of their inherent features. Trying to reduce them to something that they are not would actually be irrational and unscientific. Denying their existence because they do not fit other categories of being means dogmatically closing one's eyes to something imply because it is different. As I will try

---

174 SHESTACK. *The Philosophical Foundations…*, p. 207.
175 MACINTYRE A. *After Virtue: A Study in Moral Theory*. London: Gerald Duckworth & Co. Ltd.; 1981: p. 69.

to show, however, one can show rationally that there is an ontological foundation to human rights, and that they are therefore not in the same category as witches and unicorns.[176]

Some critics, such as Ernesto Laclau and Chantal Mouffe, have criticized a metaphysical approach to human rights as being "essentialist". In their eyes, there is no human nature as such, but only certain beliefs and values regarding it that have arisen from certain historical and cultural facts. In reality, they say, the idea that human rights are universal is a pragmatic and precarious construction.[177] This approach, however, is prone to the same criticism as the one I have tendered in the sections above, which I will not repeat here.Essentialism has a very negative connotation, for it seems to imply a speculative Platonic Heaven of Ideas. This is why Freeman prefers to speak of foundationalism or foundationalists with regard to those seeking a metaphysical basis for human rights, while I rather talk of realists seeking an ontological or metaphysical foundation.

2.3.1 The Objective Nature of the Human Person

Human Rights are based on the dignity of the human person, is my claim. I will therefore briefly discuss what defines and characterizes the human person, and thereby already shed some light on her intrinsic dignity.

The person is characterized by having a self that is incommunicable.[178] This means that she cannot lose her selfhood, even if she tried (though she can lose some of her freedom and autonomy by giving herself over to a tyrant or idol, for example). Natural elements like stones or water can be divided, diluted, set apart and brought together to form a greater whole, but the person cannot simply dissolve into a mass. Hence, Aquinas spoke about the person as never being a mere part of a whole, but always a whole of its own. Of course, human beings can stand in relationship to others (and should, as I shall show shortly), but this does not mean that they can be defined or should be treated merely with regard to this relationship. Human beings as social beings can be part of groups, regions, countries etc, but again, it is a violation to treat them as nothing but parts of a greater whole.

---

176 The fact that Christianity's anthropology is a good foundation to human rights, does not mean that they cannot be rationally argued for independently of religion or that only the believer can find a rational justification for human rights. It is true that nothing is as forceful as seeing in each human a being created in the "image of God" to respect him. Yet human dignity, as I will attempt to show, is founded in the human person independently of any religious considerations, is intelligible and therefore in principle perceivable by all.

177 LACLAU E, MOUFFE C. *Hegemony and Socialist Strategy*. English Trans. MOORE W, COMMACK P. New York: Verso; 1985: p. 153-154

178 CROSBY JF. *The Selfhood of the Human Person*. Washington: Catholic University of America Press; 1996: p. 19.

The classical definition of the human person is given by Boethius who states that a person is "an individual substance of a rational nature" (*naturæ rationalis individua substantia*). [179] By calling the person a substance, as Josef Seifert points out in his article, "Is the Right to Life or Is Another Right the Most Fundamental Human Right – The *'Urgrundrecht'?*", the implication is not that the person is merely "a thing", but rather a being standing in its own right not reducible to anything else.[180] Though the person is meant to stand in relationship to others, this does not reduce her to these relationships. Nor does the fact that the human person is embodied reduce her being to her component parts. Indeed, the substance of the person is indivisible. I cannot divide a person or turn her into multiple people.[181]

Since the human being is rational, he can in principle or at least potentially cognize the world as well as other human beings, and can also reflect on himself. The human person, as Sgreccia puts it in his magisterial work *Personalist Bioethics*, "appears above all as a *center of dynamic unification* that proceeds from within, as a unity that lasts over time, beyond all changes and beyond the psychological fluxes of a multiplicity of sensations and beyond the temporal and spatial scattering of the self". [182]

The person also possesses herself. She discovers this about herself in the experience of acting, as Karol Wojtyla argues in *The Acting Person*.[183] She possesses herself to the point that she can perform acts and is not simply driven by instincts like animals. As Damian Fedoryka points out in his article, "The Foundation of Rights in Popes John Paul II and Benedict XVI from the Perspective of the Gift", this ownership of the person, of being sui iuris also means that she determines her ultimate end. It is not contained in her nature the way it is in the grain of wheat and in the kitten to become a wheat-stalk and a full-grown cat. Rather, it is through her choices that the person decides what kind of a person she will become. Though her capacity to pose personal acts is made possiblethrough her nature, she chooses their content freely.[184]

---

179 Boethius cited in GEDDES L. *Person*. The Catholic Encyclopedia. New York; Robert Appleton Company; 1911: (accessed on 19.11.2014, at: http://www.newadvent.org/cathen/11726a.htm).

180 SEIFERT J. *Is the Right to Life or Is Another Right the Most Fundamental Human Right – The 'Urgrundrecht'?: Human Dignity, Moral Obligations, Natural Rights and Positive Law*. J East-West Thought. 2013; 3 (4): 11-31, p. 13-14. (accessed on 19.11.2014, at: http://www.csupomona.edu/ ~jet/ Documents/JET/Jet9/Seifert11-31. pdf).

181 This goes against the empiricist theories of Locke, Hume, and Parfit for example, who see in the person merely a series of successive selves and not a substance. This empiricist theory fails to acknowledge that for a being to undergo a series of successive experiences, it must be the same person having them. Otherwise, the subject cannot make sense of what he is undergoing or have a memory of what he has done or experienced. There must be something underlying these experiences, a cognizing subject, to be able to understand them, connect them and learn from them.

182SGRECCIA. *Personalist Bioethics…*, p. 137.

183 WOJTYLA K. *The Acting Person*. English Trans. POTOCKI A. Dordrecht: Reidel; 1979: p.15-16.

184 FEDORYKA D. *The Foundation of Rights in Popes John Paul II and Benedict XVI from the Perspective of the Gift*. Ave Maria Law Rev. 2012; 11 (1): 65-102, p. 74-76.

Through her choices, the person decides whether she is fundamentally turned in on herself, using the world to satisfy her needs and pleasures and emphasizing thereby her autonomy. Or she determines whether she is fundamentally turned towards the other, gives herself as a gift through love and gratefully receives from others and the world in general what she needs and what gives her joy or pleasure. In the first case, she chooses an end immanent to herself, namely her own satisfaction; in this case, the person can be explained in terms of her entelechy, the development of her own, inherent end, as Fedoryka states. In the second case, she chooses a transcendent end, an ektelechy, by giving herself as a gift to others out of love.[185]

The human person is furthermore sui iuris, as John Crosby points out in his book *The Selfhood of the Human Person*, in that human beings are never merely specimens, but are incommunicably their own. They are not merely the embodiment of an ideal of humanity, nor could they be replaced by other members of their species.[186] It is a grave violation and we experience it as such, if we are merely looked at in terms of our aesthetic qualities and intelligence, as representing a good or flawed example of the human species. The human person is furthermore sui iuris, in that she cannot be owned by another person; she possesses herself (through love, one person can be united to another – though even there she never loses herself completely).

The human person has a unique place within the universe, which is widely recognized by the natural sciences, human sciences, philosophy and many religions. Because of her capacity to know and act, the human person, contrary to animals, can therefore enter into a special relationship with the world around her. She can appreciate beauty, seek a deeper understanding of objects and the world at large from a scientific or a philosophical perspective, for example. Or, she can enter into communion with other persons in friendship or spousal love – all things that animals cannot do, since they are merely guided by their needs and instincts.[187] This is not to say that the human person is solely to be defined by her relations to the world and to others, but that they are an important aspect of her essential call and fulfillment.[188] The problem with those who think that the person is nothing but a relation, is that a substratum needs to be there in order to enter into a relationship. A pure relation cannot know and will, but a person can enter through those faculties into a relationship with others.

---

185 *Ibid.* p. 86.
186 CROSBY. *The Selfhood...*, p. 19.
187 Hence, Aristotle's definition of man as a "rational animal" does not do justice fully to the originality of his place in the cosmos, as Sgreccia points out. SGRECCIA. *Personalist Bioethics...*, p. 136. Also, the person's choice of her own end, the fact that she determines her moral nature through her choices and thus shapes herself at the very core, shows that she is more than merely a rational animal.
188 *Ibid.* p. 106, 108.

Furthermore, the human person has a body that is essential to her. One should not pretend that the body is unimportant to the human person simply because it is mortal while the soul is not.[189] It is also wrong to view the body as a machine, as Descartes thought, and therefore merely an instrument. Another version of this dualistic approach can be found in Plato who believes the body is merely the prison of the soul and should be discarded. In reality, the body belongs to the person. When I intentionally hit a person, I am not just hurting her physically, but also potentially wounding her on other levels, namely emotionally and spiritually. To dissociate her from her body is therefore artificial and goes contrary to experience.

According to the monistic theory of the neo-Marxists, as, for example, in the thought of Jean-Paul Sartre and Herbert Marcuse, however, the body is all there is of the human being and his experience. By taking back the body from bourgeois and industrial society, morality and the institution of marriage, it is turned into a place for pleasure and recreation, according to Marcuse, and becomes the starting-point for a new society. Others, like Jacques Monod, reduce human beings to their biology or, like François Jacob, to their brain. All these are variations of the reduction of the person to her body.[190]

In reality, the soul, to use Thomas Aquinas' definition, is the substantial form of the body and of the whole human being. It allows the body to carry out its activity, and is the very principle that animates it. Body and soul do not exist alongside each other, for this dualism would fail to explain the unity of activity; instead, the latter is the form of the first. "The soul", as Sgreccia puts it succinctly, "with its energy and unifying force, also activates and informs the faculties", namely rationality, will and heart that are all present in the human being at whatever stage of his development and life, even if he cannot actualize them.[191]

I conclude this discussion by pointing out that human nature has inherent and essential features that cannot be changed. One cannot turn a human person into a non-person though one can kill her and be left with a corpse. It is typical for utopians to believe that human nature can be altered, and that with time and effort, human beings will no longer need certain things like beauty, love or the truth. That she is a subject does not make her something subjective and alterable, but only highlights the fact that she has consciousness, autonomy and self-possession. Only a subject could have these features.[192] To demand that a non-subject should be able to cognize is therefore nonsensical.

---

189 For a brief synthesis of arguments for the spiritual nature of the soul and its immortality, see *Ibid*. p. 108-111.

190 For this discussion, see *Ibid*. p. 112-115.

191 *Ibid*. p. 116-7. I cannot go any further here in terms of the discussion of the relationship of soul and body, and the way the body is experienced, allows one to relate to the world, reveals the person's inner life. For a succinct overview, see *Ibid*. p. 117-122.

192 Not just totalitarian ideologies, but also certain schools of philosophy like existentialism, actualism and spiritualism think of human nature as completely open to construction. Though it is true that human beings determine their moral nature and final end through their choices, this does not mean that there is no essential nature to them. *Ibid*. p. 107.

It needs to be pointed out, however, that a definition and understanding of the human person should always refer to her dignity. She is a distinct subject because of her dignity, and I discover her preciousness precisely because it is inherent to her.[193] It is therefore somewhat artificial to distinguish between the nature of the human person and her dignity, as I have done in subdividing topics for the sake of greater clarity, for the two belong together.

2.3.2 The Dignity of the Person

According to Donnelly, there are two basic human rights theories based on human nature. The first is based on human needs, which he discards, claiming that science can only give a very restricted list of needs. The second is based on man's moral nature. Human rights are necessary to lead a life of dignity, a life worthy of the human person, and therefore arise from her intrinsic dignity.[194] The understanding of man's human nature, according to Donnelly, is based on a selection of possibilities, and combines natural social, historical and moral elements. However, Donnelly fails to give a philosophically founded anthropology and instead refers to consensus, leaving him with a circular argument.[195] He therefore does not establish philosophically what constitutes human dignity.

In his *Groundwork of the Metaphysics of Morals*, Kant speaks about human persons always having to be treated as an end; one may never use another merely as a means.[196] Even for the real or imagined good of the community, one may therefore never, for example, turn a person into a scapegoat. At the basis of this insight lies the intuition of the human person's dignity. This insight, as Josef Seifert points out, can be obtained either by looking at the structures of the person, as I have done previously. These express themselves in the following ways: through rational and intentional consciousness, the capacity to know and speak, free will and autonomy, spiritual forms of feeling, the capacity to relate to the world, to other human beings (I, Thou, We), as well as to God. Or one can gain this insight more directly by grasping the ontological basis of the essence of personhood, as we shall see.[197]

---

193 While Thomas Aquinas sees the dignity of the human person as being based on her being created in the likeness of God and therefore with freedom and rationality, one can also discover human dignity from a purely philosophical perspective, like Alexander of Hales, Rudolf Otto or Dietrich von Hildebrand did. SEIFERT. *Philosophische Grundlagen…*, p. 356-357.
194 DONNELLY. *Universal Human Rights…*, p. 16-19, 22-23.
195 FREEMAN. *The Philosophical Foundations…*, p. 503.
196 KANT I. *Kant: Groundwork of the Metaphysics of Morals*. English Trans. GREGOR MJ. Cambridge: Cambridge University Press. 1998: p. 45.
197 SEIFERT. *Is the Right to Life…*, p. 13.

The person, as I have asserted earlier, is a substance in her own right in virtue of her dignity. This dignity is an intrinsic property and an objective value that cannot be reduced to her usefulness or the manner in which she is perceived by others. She is priceless; nothing would, therefore, justify or allow her being sold into slavery or prostitution.

Following Seifert's analysis, I distinguish between four sources of human dignity. The first is the ontological dignity of the human person as such, which she has in virtue of being a human being. It is inalienable, for nothing I do can remove this dignity, though I can act against it and kill the human being. This ontological value is absolutely independent of race, age, talents, consciousness, capacities or lack thereof, simply in virtue of being a human person. This means the human being possesses this dignity independently of whether she can act or not, whether she is able to actualize her potentialities or not, and there is no gradation to human dignity.[198] This is the foundation of absolute moral obligations, expressing themselves, for example, in the basic moral principle that one should never commit an injustice neminen nocere: "To refuse to take part in committing an injustice is not only a moral duty; it is also a basic human right. Were this not so, the human person would be forced to perform an action intrinsically incompatible with human dignity, and in this way human freedom itself, the authentic meaning and purpose of which are found in its orientation to the true and the good, would be radically compromised".[199]

The second source of human dignity of the human person is based on her being conscious and rational. It arises from her capacity to actualize her rational faculties and comes to blossom in the mature person. This capacity can be lost, for example through falling into a vegetative state, and there are many degrees to it; therefore, rights arising from consciousness and rationality can also be lost. Certain rights are based on this, for example the right not to be arbitrarily deprived of consciousness (for example through "terminal sedation" at the end of life); or the right to truth, which means one's search for the truth should not be obstructed as is the case in totalitarian regimes. The right to one's own worldview is based on the human being's capacity to form a relationship with the world. The right to marriage and family is founded on the human being's capacity to form relationships. The right to religion is based on the person's capacity of transcendence and to form a relationship with God. Finally, the rights to freedom, and in particular the freedom of conscience, are founded on this source of human dignity.

The third source of human dignity is the dignity she acquires through her moral acts. It presupposes that the human being is capable of acting freely and knowing the difference between good and evil. It is not innate and can be lost through criminal behavior, for example.

---

198 *Ibid.* p. 16 ff.
199 JOHN PAUL II. *Evangelium Vitae.* (25 March 1995). Rome; 1995: §74. (accessed on 25.11.2014, at: http://www.vatican.va/holy_father/john_paul_ii/encyclicals/documents/hf_jpii_enc_25031995_evangelium-vitae_en.html).

There are different levels to it; such rights, as not to have one's reputation damaged, are grounded in it. If one loses this dignity by criminal activity, then, as a just consequence, one can be deprived, for example, of the right to freedom of movement. The particular dignity arising from choosing the good shows that the human person is called to actualize herself in this way.

The fourth source of dignity is that of a bestowed dignity. Some cases of bestowed dignity flow from interpersonal relations, such as marriage or becoming parents; others are acquired through the human community, as for example, being elected to public office. Others again, like specific talents, come from nature, while others, such as particular graces, are bestowed by God. This dignity can appear in various forms and to various degrees.

As stated earlier, human rights have to be founded on human dignity and not just on human nature as such without consideration of the person's value and dignity. If one looks at human nature without axiological considerations, then one cannot derive from it the universal right to life. One has to include human dignity to be able to do so.[200] Looking at human nature without considerations of intrinsic value, one might be tempted to follow evolutionary principles, for example, such as preferring the vital and healthy while killing the weaker.[201]

Particularly rationality and freedom are key to human dignity, especially understood as the capacity for truth (and therefore the right not to be hindered in its pursuit) and the capacity to give oneself rather than mere self-determination for the sake of doing so.[202]

2.3.3 Human Rights, Ethics and Positive Law

Human rights based on an objective and universally valid natural law became a popular theory after World War II, since it provided a basis from which Nazi criminals could be prosecuted and offered a solid foundation to combat future totalitarian human rights abuses. Since then this foundation of human rights has become much less popular. This raises the question what the relationship between human rights and morality or the natural moral law is, and what their relationship to positive law is.

---

200 Then one will come to realize the following, as Maritain so pertinently put it: "The dignity of the human person? The expression means nothing if it does not signify that by virtue of natural law, the human person has the right to be respected, is the subject of rights, possesses rights. These are things which are owed to man because of the very fact that he is man". MARITAIN J. *The Rights of Man and Natural Law*. London: The Centenary Press; 1945: p. 37.
201 SEIFERT. *Philosophische Grundlagen...*, p. 354-355.
202 *Ibid.* p. 357-359.

Moral obligations are not the same as human rights in that their field is much vaster than human rights, as Seifert points out. I have the moral obligation not to be envious of another, for example, but I am not violating another's human right by being envious of him, as long as I don't, for example, go against his right to life. Duties arise from human rights, which can and should be prosecuted by the state when violated, but this is clearly not the case regarding many moral obligations. If I fail to give my spouse the kind of warmth and attention she needs, then I am not going against her human rights, but am failing morally towards her. Furthermore, morality requires certain attitudes and inner responses, as well as the right intention. Regarding human rights, these are irrelevant, for they only consider actions. As long as I respect the human rights of others, it does not matter whether I respect somebody's right to life out fear of the law or out of love for him. However, this is crucial regarding morality.[203] Furthermore, human rights are absolute in a different sense than morality. The absoluteness of the moral law arises from a different reference-point, namely God, who issues an "ought" to me, while human rights have only other human beings as reference points. I am bound absolutely to respect the human right to life of other people, but not in the same sense as I am morally bound to God to do so.[204]

There are definitely overlaps between human rights and morality; it would be strange if this were not the case, for this would mean they pertained to an amoral or morally neutral realm. The point is rather that morality goes much further than human rights. By merely respecting human rights, I am not yet a morally good person, for I might be missing the intentions and attitudes which are essential to a morally good act.[205]

Human rights, which concern fundamental goods like the right to life, are different from positive law though the latter should reflect it, mainly in the constitution of a state. When positive law does not respect them, as is the case in totalitarian regimes, then one can see the difference between positive law and human rights clearly. Ideally speaking, positive law should reflect human rights, but it can never be their ultimate source.

As Seifert points out, there are some rights which are absolute like the right to life and some which are relative or "relational rights" that arise only vis-à-vis certain human beings, for example of children towards their parents.[206] But we've already looked at this in the section on the distinction between the fourfold source of human dignity.

---

203 SEIFERT. *Is the Right to Life…*, p. 21-22.
204 *Ibid.* p. 23-24.
205 However, Seifert goes a different path from other "foundationalists", as Freeman would term them, in basing human rights on the four-fold sources of dignity of the human person, while others would ground them on the natural law (i.e. morality) arising from God as well as the dignity of the human person. It seems to me that one can bring both together, by pointing out that since moral oughts are present when it comes to authentic human rights, one is both called to respect the right to life of another because of his human right, but also because of the absolute ought issued to me by God through morality. To discuss this point further would, however, go beyond the scope of this dissertation.
206 *Ibid.*

As a working definition of human rights, I would therefore suggest the following: basic human rights are universal claims on others to standards of behavior rooted in every human being's dignity. Basic human rights should be legally enforceable, are universally valid, innate and inalienable. They can only be derogated from in exceptional circumstances depending on the norm's intrinsic importance and its position in the hierarchy of rights. This brings me to the next point, namely the question if there exists a hierarchy of rights.

2.4 A Hierarchy of Rights

There is an inherent problem with every human being having many legally actionable rights. It is inevitable that conflicts between rights will arise and eventually need to be resolved by laws and in the courts. But attempting to establish a hierarchy of human rights is controversial.[207] Courts, particularly international human rights tribunals, are increasingly faced with the difficult task of deciding which rights take precedence.[208] My purpose is to argue for a prioritization among human rights as intellectually defensible and also ultimately a workable approach in bioethics when the pursuit of different rights inevitably produces clashes.

2.4.1 A Historical Overview of the Legal Debate: Problems and Contradictions

The OHCHR and the UN in general reject the notion of any hierarchy of human rights, and in particular that economic, social and cultural rights have a "second-class" status behind civil and political rights.[209] "All human rights are universal, indivisible and interdependent and interrelated. The international community must treat human rights globally in a fair and equal manner, on the same footing, and with the same emphasis".[210] At the same time, one sees several important caveats both in the Vienna Declaration and Programme of Action and positions emanating from the OHCHR. The VDPA states that different cultural, religious

---

207 KLEIN E. *Establishing a Hierarchy of Human Rights: Ideal Solution or Fallacy?*. Isr Law Rev. 2008; 41: 477-488.

208 SHELTON D. *Hierarchy of Norms and Human Rights: Of Trumps and Winners*. Sask Law Rev. 2002; 65: 301-331.

209 UNITED NATIONS COMMITTEE ON ECONOMIC, SOCIAL AND CULTURAL RIGHTS. *Fact Sheet No.16*. (REV.1). Geneva: OHCR; 1995 (accessed on 22.11.2014, at: http://www.ohchr.org/ Documents/ Publications/FactSheet16rev.1en.pdf).

210 WORLD CONFERENCE ON HUMAN RIGHTS. *Vienna Declaration…*, § 5.

backgrounds and national particularities "must be borne in mind" as states fulfill the duty to promote and protect all human rights.[211]

The OHCHR states that "no human right is intrinsically inferior to any other. A certain right can still be given priority, but only on practical grounds—e.g., because it has historically been neglected or is likely to act as a catalyst".[212] Nevertheless, the list of OHCHR accepted reasons for human rights not to be equally enforced or promoted continue to mount. "Human rights law recognizes that a lack of resources can impede the realization of human rights. Accordingly, some human rights obligations are of a progressive kind, while others are immediate."[213] The OHCHR recognizes that certain internationally recognized human rights may be limited to preserve "public order" or "public health" and even "can lawfully be derogated from, or suppressed, in times of public emergencies, such as a security crisis", but other human rights that are basic to immediate human survival may never be derogated from.[214] This last example is so evident an example of a recognized real difference in importance among human rights that it makes the OHCHR's firm denial of any human rights ranking earlier in the same document puzzling. Teraya Koji argues that the existence of non-derogable rights shows that a hierarchy clearly exists among human rights.[215]

Navi Pillay, when she served as UN High Commissioner for Human Rights, wrote the following with reference to the deposit of the 10th ratification instrument, by the government of Uruguay, of the Optional Protocol of the International Covenant on Economic, Social and Cultural Rights. "More than sixty years ago, the Universal Declaration of Human Rights promised universality, indivisibility and equal value of all human rights for all people. Its drafters wisely chose not to rank rights. On the contrary, they recognized that civil and political rights go hand in hand with economic, social and cultural rights. Yet, for far too long economic, social and cultural rights were not given the same attention and status in law, lagging behind on means for promotion and protection, as well as resources, when compared to civil and political rights".[216]

---

211 *Ibid.*

212 OFFICE OF THE UNITED NATIONS HIGH COMMISSIONER FOR HUMAN RIGHTS (OHCHR). *Frequently Asked Questions on a Human Rights-Based Approach to Development Cooperation.* New York: OHCR; 2006: p. 11. (accessed on 19.11.2014, at: http://www.ohchr.org/Documents/Publications/FAQen. pdf).

213 *Ibid.* p. 2.

214 *Ibid.* p. 3.

215 KOJI T. *Emerging Hierarchy in International Human Rights and Beyond: From the Perspective of Nonderogable Rights,* Eur J Int Law. 2001; 12: 917-941.

216 PILLAY N. *Statement by Navi Pillay, the UN High Commissioner for Human Rights at the deposit of the 10th ratification instrument, by Uruguay, of the Optional Protocol of the International Covenant on Economic, Social and Cultural Rights, delivered by Assistant Secretary-General for Human Rights Ivan Šimonović* (6 February 2013). New York; 2013 (accessed on 20.11.2014, at: http://www.ohchr.org/EN/NewsEvents/Pages/ DisplayNews.aspx?NewsID= 12971&LangID=E).

Pillay recognizes that economic, social and cultural rights were not seen as equal to civil and political rights in the recent past. Actually, the OHCHR would seem to accept the inferiority of economic, social and cultural rights themselves, notwithstanding declarations to the contrary... They say States must only ensure an "essential minimum" of economic, social and cultural rights and their "progressive realization" while States have "core obligations" derived from such rights as those to life and food, which are "binding constraints" that "cannot be traded off." [217] This is another example showing that some rights "cannot be derogated from" while others may indeed be justifiably suppressed or not prioritized for a variety of reasons.

I contend that to assert the absolute equality of the very long list of internationally recognized human rights is utopian and leads to immediate difficulties and even deadlock as soon as these human rights conflict. Unacceptable outcomes are the logical consequence of the "all human rights are absolutely equal" position. For example, no decisive action could be taken when one human's right to private property comes into conflict with another's right to food. Taken to its absolute extreme, this position would mean a persons' right to freedom of movement would prohibit any form of incarceration/quarantine and would be more compatible with a state of anarchy than with a well ordered society. Many of these extreme cases can be resolved by acknowledging that no, or at least very few, human rights may not be lawfully circumscribed and limited. Acknowledging that some rights may indeed be severely limited and even derogated from while others may not, however, is already a significant step towards ranking human rights.[218]

It is perhaps understandable that subsidiary bodies of the United Nations Organization should refuse to acknowledge openly a hierarchy among recognized human rights, since the UN has failed to hammer out such a ranking. The UN is notorious for its long negotiations often ending in failure to achieve consensus on many issues. It has also been said to "suffer from occasional mindless extravagance" when drafting human rights.[219] In practice, however, even at the UN, certain rights like the right to life clearly have ascendancy over "lesser" rights or rights derived from more fundamental rights as we noted above in the OHCHR's own words.

There is furthermore a modern problem of "rights inflation", where more and more rights are claimed with the added problem that they come into conflict with other recognized rights. James Griffin makes the point well. "The belief is widespread that human rights mark what is most important in morality; so whatever any group in society regards as most important, it will be strongly tempted to declare to be a human right".[220] Having something declared to be a human right is a way to push it powerfully towards becoming a legal right, but this has had the unfortunate side effect of debasing the term human right.[221] The alternatives are either

---

217 OHCHR. *Frequently Asked Questions...*, p. 12.
218 SHELTON. *Hierarchy of Norms...*, p. 316.
219 GRIFFIN J. *On Human Rights*. Oxford: Oxford University Press; 2013: p. 292 endnote 8.
220 *Ibid.* p. 92.
221 *Ibid.*

a deadlocked situation between contending human rights, or de facto prioritizing between rights while hypocritically denying it as the UN does, or attempting to elucidate at least some prioritization among rights as courts can be forced to do when making rulings.

2.4.2 The Philosophical Basis for a Hierarchy of Rights

The most foundational source for human rights is human dignity as it arises from the human person's essential capacity for self-possession and self-transcendence, as I have shown previously. Hence, only those goods that are central to the life and good of the human person can be at the basis of human rights.[222] Others, such as the "right to internet", for example, are too external to the core concerns of a person to be authentic human rights. Therefore, the centrality of goods to the welfare of the human person also determine their hierarchical important. Furthermore, Seifert's distinction between different kinds of dignity also determines the order of importance regarding the rights flowing from them. Both the rights to life and conscience have a claim to being the most fundamental human rights. This is so because the right to life stems from the ontological dignity of the human person and is the answer to the question: "Which right refers to the most basic good that is the condition of all others?"[223] "The enjoyment of the right to life is a necessary condition of the enjoyment of all other human rights".[224] On the other hand, the rights to respect for conscience and to religious freedom are higher ranked rights in one sense since only living without anything added is not the highest good for a human person.[225] For rational and conscious agents, conscience and religion are the highest values linked to free will and thus could also be called the most fundamental human rights.[226]

2.5 Concrete Example of Human Rights Conflicts in Health Care

Having shown how a case can be made for the right to life and the right to conscience as the most fundamental human rights, we turn to some more concrete examples of the resolution of some cases of human rights conflicts. A modern example came during the 2002/2003 Severe Acute Respiratory Syndrome (SARS) epidemic, when numerous quarantines restricted the movements of persons infected or possibly infected with SARS in the name of

---

222 SEIFERT. *Philosophische Grundlagen*...p. 250.
223 SEIFERT. *Is the Right to Life*..., p. 27.
224 PRZETACZNIK F. *The Right to Life as a Basic Human Right*. Hum Rights J. 1976; 9: 589-603. p. 589.
225 SEIFERT. *Is the Righ to Life*..., p. 29.
226 *Ibid.*

public health concerns, specifically the rights to life and health of others.[227] These quarantines were generally accepted, but in the case of Acquired Immune Deficiency Syndrome (AIDS) quarantine of infected individuals has been almost universally rejected for a number of practical and ethical reasons.[228] It remains a generally accepted principle, however, that when faced with epidemics of life-threatening infectious diseases, public authorities may impose quarantines that do curtail certain rights, freedom of movement and association, in favor of other rights that are deemed more fundamental, principally the right to life.

2.6 Consequences of Denying a Hierarchy of Rights

It is interesting to examine the thorny ethical questions of conscience rights in the health care field by looking at the results when conscience rights are overruled. In the absence of conclusive proof that another human right trumps conscience rights in these cases, all that remains is a raw "might makes right" ethics prejudicial to objecting health workers. This domination of the stronger party over the weaker is the antithesis of the basic concepts underlying human rights, essentially that universally human beings have equal rights and that any form of coercion in denying the exercise of a human right must be justified with the strongest arguments.

An isolated example is Sweden, one of the very few countries that make no provision for the conscience rights of health care personnel.[229] In practice, most medical personnel must be prepared to carry out any legal procedure which they are ordered to perform or face legal sanctions and in short order dismissal from employment or even employability in the medical field if they refuse in conscience to participate. The right to professional conscientious objection is denied to medical workers by the Swedish State in a manner more reminiscent of authoritarian regimes than of democratic human rights respecting states and has resulted in an official complaint being filed at the Council of Europe's European Committee of Social Rights.[230] Their national parliament went so far as to vote on 11 May 2011 to approve a foreign affairs committee report vowing to work internationally against a 2010 resolution by the

227 Generally speaking, legal systems accept the violation of what are regarded as lesser rights if that is done as a necessary means for preventing the violation of more fundamental rights. XIAOBING X, WILSON G. *On Conflict of Human Rights*. Pierce Law Rev. 2006; 5 (1): 31-57, p. 32.
228 LEWIN T. *Rights of Citizens and Society Raise Legal Muddle on AIDS*. New York Times (14 October 1987) New York; 1987: p. A1.
229 KISKA R. *Sweden's Aggressive Attack on Conscience Challenged Before the Council of Europe*. Zenit (14 June 2014). Rome; 2014 (accessed on 19.11.2014, at: http: //www.zenit.org/en/articles/sweden-saggressive-attack-on-conscience-challenged-before-the-council-of-europe).
230 *Ibid.*

Parliamentary Assembly of the Council of Europe in favor of conscience rights in the health care field.[231]

Such harsh measures are hard to explain when taken by liberal democracies that self identify as protectors of an ever-expansive number of personal liberties and rights. Forcing medical personnel to violate their deeply held beliefs contradicts the cherished liberal principle that everyone should be free to think and act as they wish with only minimal restrictions on what they can or cannot do.

2.6.1 Objections to Conscience Rights

An obstacle for the acceptance of conscientious objection is the argument that health sector workers have professional obligations that trump their ethical beliefs and rights.[232] The most persuasive version of this argument is the so-called "gatekeeper" view.[233] Succinctly put, medical professionals in many modern societies have been granted a legal monopoly over certain services/products in exchange for subsidized professional training and a willingness to make these services/products available to the general public with a high standard of safety. If a doctor refuses to perform, for example, an abortion, the monopolistic system can in some circumstances make it difficult or impossible for a person to access the procedure. Less stringent versions of this position would not require a medical professional to participate actively in a procedure he/she finds morally repulsive, but do find it reasonable to force him/her to refer patients to another practitioner who is willing to provide the service.[234] It remains hard to see how any such "compromise" is reasonable when one is demanding that a medical professional accept a violation of his/her recognized human right to conscience when other means of resolving the conflict can be found such as having 24 hour medical referral services available through call centers or online. It is, however, eminently reasonable to require doctors, or other medical practitioners, to declare immediately their conscientious objection to certain procedures that are generally available to assist potential patients.

Certainly, the most serious objection to physicians exercising their conscience rights and refusing to cooperate in certain procedures is the counterclaim that the patient's human rights are being violated. Should the human right not to be forced to violate one's conscience be valued at a lower level than the right to access medical services or the rights of autonomous

231 SWEDISH PARLIAMENT. *Freedom of Conscience in Health Care* (11 May 2011). Stockholm; 2011 (accessed on 19.11.2014, at: http://www.consciencelaws.org/background/society/society004.aspx).
232 SAVULESCU J. *Conscientious Objection in Medicine*. Br Med J. 2006; 332: 294-297.
233 CANTOR JD. *Conscientious Objection Gone Awry: Restoring Selfless Professionalism in Medicine*. N Engl J Med. 2009; 360 (15): 1484-1485.
234 WICCLAIR MR. *Conscientious Objection in Medicine*. Bioethics. 2000; 14 (3): 205-227, p. 218.

choice of patients? The latter assertion is paradoxical, since the very same right to autonomy of the health care worker/s is being denied in order to accommodate the patient's autonomy.[235] These ethical problems of conflicting rights become particularly problematic, when one of two people wants his/her right recognized to the exclusion of the same right for the other. The classic formulation of the right to autonomy I have cited before as, "your right to swing your arms ends just where the other man's nose begins", shows the inherent contradiction of this position.[236] I agree with Beauchamp and Childress when they say, "A patient's right of autonomy should not be purchased at the price of the physician's parallel right".[237] The view that the autonomy ofpatients should overrule the autonomy of medical professionals places significant burdens, since the person seeking a procedure generally has alternative providers to safeguard his/her autonomy, but health workers only have the options of resigning from their profession or losing their autonomy and sacrificing their right of conscience. It is true that physicians in particular have professional responsibilities that limit their autonomy, but these cannot override such ethical principles as the protection of life, of the physical and psychological health of human beings, the need to provide pain relief and respect for the freedom and dignity of the human person.[238]

2.7 Ways to Resolve Human Rights Conflicts in the Medical Field

This leaves the important question of which recognized right, that of access to health services or of conscience should prevail? One ethical principle that is especially useful in these dilemmas is the general norm that "negative rights" take precedence over "positive rights" in most cases.[239] This principle is based on the observation that, for example, violating the negative version of the right to life, the right not to be actively killed, is more often prosecuted and bears greater social stigma than violating the positive version of the right to life, which would include such omissions as not providing life-sustaining food, water, shelter, medical care, etc.[240]

---

235 REQUENA P. *Un Paradosso della bioetica Nordamericana: Autonomia vs. Conscienza.* Acta Philosophica. 2011; 20 (1): 167-171, p. 171.

236 CHAFFEE. *Freedom of Speech...*, p. 957.

237 BEAUCHAMP T, CHILDRESS J. *Principles of Biomedical Ethics.* New York: Oxford University Press; 20015: p. 38.

238 SACCHINI D, ANTICO L. *The Professional Autonomy of the Medical Doctor in Italy.* Theor Med Bioeth. 2000; 21 (5): 441-456, p. 442.

239 WEBER E. *Positive and Negative Rights: What's the Difference, and Why Does It Matter?* (2 May 2009). San Francisco; 2009 (accessed on 27.08.2014, at: http://everyday-ethics.org/positive-and-negativerights-whats-the-difference-and-why-does-it-matter/).

240 This is especially true regarding strangers or individuals towards whom a person has no special duties or responsibilities. Forcibly preventing a person from accessing food, water, etc. however, can be seen as actively killing or violating the negative right to life.

The influential Czech jurist Karel Vasak divided human rights into "three generations". [241] A case can be made for a hierarchy ranking first generation rights, i.e. negative rights in the civil and political arena, highest. The argument is essentially that these rights areessential for the life and dignity of human persons and can be respected even with minimal resources available. Second generation rights favor equality such as free universal elementary education and are positive rights which can be seen as ranking lower.[242] Third generation rights are still ill defined but are generally seen as even less important/enforceable as they go beyond recognized civil and social rights in such directions as self-determination, collective rights, natural resource preservation for "future generations", etc.[243] The three generations classification corresponds loosely to the French governmental motto: "*Liberté, égalité, fraternité*".[244]

Many accept that human rights were recognized chronologically in "three generations", but insist that this does not imply precedence for first generation human rights over second or third generation rights.[245] Others argue that the very doctrine of human rights having universal application is the imposition of a hierarchy based on Western values.[246]

A problem with this position is that it does not explain satisfactorily why certain rights were intuitively and almost universally recognized first. Nor does it provide an answer to the practical problem of prioritizing the safeguarding of human rights, except by the use of misleading language as employed by the UN's OHCHR. To speak plainly, disaster relief begins with saving human lives in immediate peril and then proceeds down a hierarchical path of services until other human rights such as education and freedom of speech are finally assured.

There are many "real world" implications flowing from how human rights are ranked. A persuasive argument can be made that the negative right to life, i.e. not to be actively killed, is the highest in the pantheon of human rights. This assertion is usually supported by the argument that other recognized rights, such as freedom of speech, are dependent for their effective exercise on the prior right to life. Along with the right to life, the rights to freedom of thought, conscience and religion have been ranked at the top of human rights included in the 1948 Universal Declaration along with the prohibitions against torture and slavery as rights from which no derogation is permitted under the binding ICCPR.[247]

---

241 WELLMAN C. *Solidarity, the Individual and Human Rights.* Hum Rights Q. 2000; 22: 639-657, p. 639.
242 Diego Gracia argues that these rights are really moral rights deriving from moral obligations which create lower level human rights. GRACIA GUILLÉN D. *Fondamenti di Bioetica: Sviluppo Storico e Metodo.* Italian Trans. FELICIANI AJ, SPINSANTI S.Milan: Edizioni San Paolo; 1993: p. 316.
243 *Ibid.*
244 "Liberty, Equality, Fraternity".

245 KLEIN. *Establishing a Hierarchy...*, p. 480.
246 KOSKENNIEMI M. *Hierarchy in International Law: A Sketch.* Eur J Int Law. 1997; 8: 566-582, p. 582.
247 QUEENSLAND PUBLIC INTEREST LAW CLEARING HOUSE INC. (QPILCH). *The Hierarchy of Human Rights.* QPILCH Database, Brisbane (accessed on 28.09.2014, at: http://www.qpilch.org.au/_dbase_upl/E_Human Rights.pdf).

Historical observations support a high ranking for conscience rights. Extraordinary numbers of people throughout the ages have made tremendous sacrifices to safeguard their right to freedom of conscience, frequently in the form of religious freedom. Entire populations have gone into exile rather than accept forced conversion. Christian and other martyrs, when faced with the stark alternatives of death or violating their consciences, opted to maintain their beliefs rather than their lives. Socrates is perhaps the most famous example from ancient times. His argument was that it is a far worse to do evil than to endure it to be done to oneself.[248]

The new category of organizations founded specifically to defend human rights historically came into existence to protest the sufferings of the distinct category of "prisoners of conscience" generally persecuted by authoritarian and totalitarian regimes.[249] Conscience rights clearly command respect and are among the short list of values/rights for which large numbers have been willing to die over the centuries.

It is astonishing that in a few modern societies the positive "right to access health care" of an individual is determined to justify coercing the negative conscience rights of a health care worker. Sometimes these are the legal legacies of totalitarian systems such as communist regimes, but some of the worst offenders are liberal democracies that self identify as champions of human rights. The right to access health care is clearly a second generation positive right, since the emphasis is on equality of access, while not being coerced into performing a procedure that goes against one's conscience is a first generation negative right. A strong argument can therefore be made that these kinds of conscience rights, not to be forced to actively violate one's conscience, should take precedence and prevail.

There are serious legal issues when human rights come into conflict. This problem is further complicated by a lack of consensus concerning prioritization among human rights. Nevertheless, a solid legal and ethical case can be made that the right to life should trump other human rights claims, particularly in its negative version. I believe that there is a strong logic to prioritizing the three generations of human rights as generally more important to less so. Viewing the problem of conscience conflicts in health care settings through the prism of conflicting rights and attempting to determine which rights should prevail is a helpful exercise. I concur with the generally high position that the human right of conscience of health care professionals, generally in the form of conscientious objection, has been granted in most legislation, court cases and ethical reflection on the issue as we will see in the following chapters.

---

248 PLATO. *Plato's Gorgias...*, p. 38.
249 Amnesty International is perhaps the most famous of these groups.

CHAPTER 3:

ANALYSIS OF CONSCIENCE CONFLICTS

There are various ways of dealing with legal obligations that go against one's conscience as a health care provider. Today, we are most familiar with conscientious objection, but this has been a relatively recent legal development. I will give a historical overview in this chapter, as well as differentiating conscientious objection from other means of resistance, namely conscientious subversion and civil disobedience. Conscientious objection, as I will show, provides a kind of witness that is uniquely suited to the medical profession in protecting it from going against the Hippocratic Oath. The goal is not to give medical health professionals arbitrary power to decide what they will or will not do, which would put in danger the health of their patients, but to discern clearly which guidelines will protect both them as well as the people in their care. To oblige doctors to go against their conscience is a dangerous policy. As patients we know that the skills of health workers can save us, but if their principles are flawed, we will be less willing to put our lives into their hands. For if they have violated their consciences in some cases, what prevents them from doing so again, especially if they no longer see their profession as exclusively defending and preserving life?

3.1 Conscientious Subversion

Conscientious subversion occurs when a person has a conscientious conflict but chooses not to make this known publicly and does not openly refrain from participating in a medical practice of which she disapproves, but instead acts to circumvent the purposes for which the law or regulation exists.[250] It is interesting to note that the very first medical conscience issue recorded in history involved conscientious subversion. The Hebrew midwives were morally opposed to carrying out Pharaoh's orders to kill newborn boys, but they did not express their refusal openly. Instead, they pretended to cooperate and made up an excuse for not committing the infanticides. "So the king of Egypt summoned the midwives and asked them, 'Why have you done this, allowing the boys to live?' The midwives answered Pharaoh, 'The Hebrew women are not like the Egyptian women. They are robust and give birth before the midwife arrives'".[251]

---

250 JANSEN L. *HIV Exceptionalism, CD4+ Cell Testing, and Conscientious Subversion.* J Med Ethics. 2005; 31 (6): 322-326, p. 324.
251 EXODUS 1:18-19.

Clearly, the main ethical issues surrounding conscientious subversion is the use of deception and even outright lying that frequently accompanies this practice as well as material cooperation with evil. These ethical problems prevented John Locke from openly embracing the concept, although he hinted at it as a tactic in his writing.[252] A major predicament for persons with conscientious objections in the ancient and even relatively modern world was the enormous personal cost of standing up in conscience to political/religious authorities when refusing to cooperate with evil. It was common practice for conscientious objectors literally to lose their heads.

Thomas More walked a fine line between conscientious subversion and conscientious objection. He tried to avoid openly expressing his conflict of conscience, but he also refused to have any part in unethical cooperation with anything his conscience would not permit. More's case is valuable and edifying from several points of view. He showed clearly that the praiseworthy ethical act of refusing to submit to an unjust legal requirement is not the fruit of a haughty decision on the part of someone who puts him/herself above the law. He did not rebel against King Henry VIII, but he steadfastly refused to swear falsely the oath declaring the king to be the Supreme Head of the Church in England. The heart of the matter was coherence with one's own fundamental values: "My case was such in this matter through the clearness of my own conscience that though I might have pain I could not have harm, for a man may in such a case lose his head and not have harm".[253] He refused to lie or perjure himself and this commitment to the truth and his judgment of conscience eventually led to his execution.

By its very nature it is difficult to ascertain how common conscientious subversion is in the health care professions. There is, however, substantial anecdotal evidence of such actions as "slow codes" or "Hollywood codes" where health workers who are required to perform re-animation on patients in cardiac arrest, but who do not think it is the proper course of action, respond slowly and without enthusiasm so as to maximize the chances of the intervention failing.[254] The American College of Physicians ethics manual mentions and condemns "slow codes" as deceptive and therefore unethical.[255] Another example is when a pharmacist lies and tells a client the pharmacy is "out" of morningafter pills to avoid selling them.

---

252 DUNN J. *The Political Thought of John Locke: An Historical Account of the Argument of the 'Two Treatises of Government.* Cambridge: Cambridge University Press; 1982. p. 34

253 MORE T. *Letter to Margaret Roper from the Tower of London* (June 3, 1535). London; 1535 (accessed on 25.10.2014, at: http://www.thomasmorestudies.org/quotes.html).

254 JONSEN AR, SIEGLER M, WINSLADE WJ. *Un Approccio Pratico alle Decisioni Etiche inMedicina Clinica.* Italian Trans. FALLANI A. SPAGNOLO AG (editor). Milan: The McGraw Hill Companies, Inc.; 2003: p. 46.

255 SNYDER L. *American College of Physicians Ethics Manual:* Sixth Edition. Ann Intern Med. 2012; 156 (1_Part_2): 73-104, p. 84.

The Bible offers us the example of the scribe Eleazar who refused to save himself with an act of conscientious subversion where he would pretend to eat pork. He preferred to die than to risk scandalizing particularly the young Jews and running the risk that others would eat pork, thinking they were following his example.[256] I concur that conscientious objection, or when this is not allowed, civil disobedience are more acceptable means of resolving conflicts of conscience in the health care arena. Conscientious subversion is a tactic that lacks the honesty and witness value that are strengths of conscientious objection and civil disobedience. It can only be ethically justified in rare circumstances when authorities are highly oppressive and if the person does not actively do what her conscience forbids. Conscientious subversion can furthermore very easily lead to the undermining of public confidence in the reliability and honesty of health professionals.

3.2 Civil Disobedience

Civil disobedience involves the illegal refusal to obey certain laws or regulations as a protest because they are deemed unjust and violate the objector's conscience. Punishment for this disobedience is expected but seen as part of the effective resistance to the injustice. Martin Luther King Jr. famously wrote on this subject, "I submit that an individual who breaks a law that conscience tells him is unjust, and who willingly accepts the penalty of imprisonment in order to arouse the conscience of the community over its injustice, is in reality expressing the highest respect for law".[257] The idea that there can be a duty to disobey unjust laws has a distinguished pedigree. Thomas Aquinas summed up a long tradition of scholarship on the topic. "I answer that, As Augustine says (De Lib. Arb. i, 5) 'that which is not just seems to be no law at all': wherefore the force of a law depends on the extent of its justice. Now in human affairs a thing is said to be just, from being right, according to the rule of reason. But the first rule of reason is the law of nature, as is clear from what has been stated above (91, 2, ad 2). Consequently every human law has just so much of the nature of law, as it is derived from the law of nature. But if in any point it deflects from the law of nature, it is no longer a law but a perversion of law".[258]

Civil disobedience's popularity as a term can be traced back to an essay by Henry David Thoreau, who in turn was influenced by a poem of Percy Shelley, "The Masque of Anarchy". Thoreau refused to pay taxes that would be used to support the Mexican American War or the institution of slavery and in consequence was imprisoned for a night. "It costs me less

---

256 2 Maccabees 6: 18-31.
257 KING ML Jr. *Letter from Birmingham Jail* (16 April 1963) Birmingham: 1963 (accessed on 21.10.2014, at: http://www.africa.upenn.edu/Articles_Gen/Letter_Birmingham.html).
258 AQUINAS. *Summa Theologica…*, I-II, q. 95. a. 2.

in every sense to incur the penalty of disobedience to the State than it would to obey".[259] His philosophical and practical perspective influenced several subsequent important civil disobedience leaders.

Arguably, the most famous civil disobedience leader was Mohandas Ghandi who adopted the term used by Thoreau to explain his actions to English readers, but he arrived at his program of action after studying his Hindu religious texts.[260] He became the primary leader in the decades long protest movement which led to Indian independence from Great Britain. His movement stressed non-violence as part of a philosophy of life he called Satyagraha that seeks to confront might with love, non-violence and suffering.[261] Ghandi's insistence on non-violent civil disobedience to touch the consciences of oppressors and observers had a profound impact on such leaders such as Martin Luther King Jr. who used civil disobedience in their movements.

Civil disobedience is inherently a political act and therefore is more a strategy of protest than one commonly associated with health care workers. In extreme circumstances, however, doctors and other health workers have used civil disobedience. Almost the entire corps of Dutch medical doctors actively refused to cooperate with the occupying authorities during World War II when asked to perform unethical acts such as identifying persons for euthanasia. Most Dutch physicians lost their right to practice publicly medicine and one hundred doctors were imprisoned in concentration camps with many losing their lives as punishment for this act of civil disobedience.[262] The Rescue movement in the United States shook the health care sector with over 60,000 arrests just in the period 1988-1993 in civil disobedience sit-ins blocking access to abortion centers.[263] Some doctors and nurses participated, but generally speaking protestors were not health care workers.

During the Nuremberg "Doctors Trials" in 1946 and 1947, there was repeated mention that German physicians failed in their conscientious duty to resist the unethical demands of the NAZI regime.[264] The "Nuremberg defense" that unethical acts were done "just following orders" was decisively rejected. They were condemned by the tribunal for failing to exercise

---

259 THOREAU HD. *Civil Disobedience.* (Original Title: Resistance to Civil Government) Concord; 1849 (accessed on 20.10.2014, at: http://www.transcendentalists.com/civil_disobedience.htm).

260 WEBER T. *Gandhi as Disciple and Mentor.* Cambridge: Cambridge University Press; 2004: p. 44.

261 SAVITA S, GANDHI M, GANDHI S, *ET AL. Satyagraha.* New Delhi: Publications Division, Indian Ministry of Information and Broadcasting; 2007: p. 23.

262 ALEXANDER. *Medical Science under Dictatorship...*, p. 45.

263 CAVANAUGH-O'KEEFE J. *Pro-Life Movement In The United States* in TIERNEY H (editor). *Women's Studies Encyclopedia.* Westport: Greenwood Press; 2002 (accessed on 25.11.2014, at: http://gem.greenwood.com/wse/wsePrint.jsp?id=id538).

264 TAYLOR. *Opening Statement...*, (accessed on 25.10.2014, at: http://law2.umkc.edu/faculty/projects/ftrials/nuremberg/doctoropen.html).

their duty to refuse to obey orders or laws that gravely violated human rights even if technically "legal" under the laws of the Third Reich. The International Law Commission stated that "the fact that a person acted pursuant to an order of his Government or of a superior d[id]… not relieve him from responsibility under international law, provided a moral choice was in fact possible to him".[265] The guidelines created for what constitutes a war crime became known as the "Nuremberg Principles" and set an important precedent in international law that can be invoked to support civil disobedience in the health care field.

Civil disobedience finds its ethical justification in the right to disobey and protest unjust laws or regulations. When it is strictly nonviolent, this characteristic reduces the ethical problems associated with protests that break the law. Nevertheless, civil disobedience is a very serious action since it involves rejecting the authority of the law which is necessary for preserving the common good. "Authority is before all else a moral force. For this reason the appeal of rulers should be to the individual conscience, to the duty which every man has of voluntarily contributing to the common good".[266] This can be justified when all other suitable means of peaceful protest and civil actions failed to yield results.[267] It remains especially ethically problematic to carry out acts of civil disobedience in the health care field, however, since a less extreme form of conscience protection exists for most health professionals, namely conscientious objection.

3.3 Conscientious Objection

3.3.1 Characteristics

The word objection comes from the Latin verb objicere ("to throw against").[268] Conscientious objection can be defined as refusing to comply with an authoritative order or rule because this directive violates another fundamental ethical obligation. In other words, conscientious objection can be the act of refusing to obey a civil law believed in conscience to be gravely unjust.[269] We know that conscientious objection, in a strict sense, was theoretically and legally

265 UNITED NATIONS INTERNATIONAL LAW COMMISSION. *Principles of International…*, (accessed on 25.10.2014, at: http://legal.un.org/ilc/texts/instruments/english/draft%20articles/7_1_1950.pdf).

266 JOHN XXIII. *Pacem in Terris*. (11 April 1963). Rome; 1963: § 48. (accessed on 20.11.2014, at: http://www.vatican.va/holy_father/john_xxiii/encyclicals/documents/hf_jxxiii_enc_11041963_pacem_en.html).

267 SÁEZ CABRERA C. *La Desobedencia Civil*. Anuario de Derechos Humanos. Nueva Época. 2000; 1: 311-355. p. 320.

268 LIVERANI PG. *Coscienza o Autodeterminazione?* in LIVERANI PG (editor). *L'Obiezione di Coscienza tra Libertà e Responsabilità*. Siena: Cantagalli; 2013: 119-121, p. 120.

269 CARRASCO DE PAOLA I, PENNACCHINI M. *Coscienza* in SGRECCIA E, TARANTINO A (editors). *Enciclopedia di Bioetica e Scienza Giuridica: Vol. III Cadavere-Cyborg*. Naples: Edizioni Scientifiche Italiane; 2010: 679-689, p. 682.

defined only recently, a little over a century ago, first regarding the refusal to bear and use weapons in a military context. The reality of people refusing to violate their consciences even when facing grave penalties, however, appears to have always existed.[270] Conscientious objection differs from civil disobedience in that the objector is necessarily personally involved in the problematic situation and does not seek by his/her refusal to make a political protest which breaks the law. Conscientious objectors, in fact, expect legal protection of their right not to be forced to participate in actions they deem morally reprehensible.

Conscientious objection in the health care field, a refusal to participate or cooperate by a medical professional when a procedure violates his/her conscience that is protected by law, has become a growing practical concern for legislators and a source of contentious debates among ethicists and the general public.[271] The practice of conscientious objection in medicine is widely recognized and regulated in laws and regulations. Indeed, the massive growth of conscientious objection in recent decades occurred after the legalization in many countries of abortion and, in a few modern cases, euthanasia and legalization in many countries of abortion and, in a few modern cases, euthanasia and assisted suicide, which created new professional requirements for health care professionals and grave ethical conflicts for many.[272]

As discussed in chapter two, conscience rights are recognized as important basic human rights. It is, however, necessary to make a distinction between conscience rights in general and the right of conscientious objection in particular. Freedom of conscience and religion are foundational values in pluralistic legal systems, while the right to conscientious objection must be balanced with other constitutional values and prevented from being invoked unjustifiably or indiscriminately.[273] It should be axiomatic, however, that recognized rights to conscience must safeguard not just beliefs but also accompanying manifestations of conduct.[274]

---

270 LAFFITTE J. *Storia dell'Obiezione di Coscienza e Differenti Accezioni del Concetto di Tolleranza* in SGRECCIA E, LAFFITTE J (editors). *La Coscienza Christiana a Sostegno del Diritto alla Vita.* Rome: Libreria Editrice Vaticana; 2008: 112-139, p. 112.

271 ALTA CHARO R. *The Celestial Fire of Conscience — Refusing to Deliver Medical Care.* N Eng J Med. 2005; 352: 2471-2473; WICCLAIR MR. *Is Conscientious Objection Incompatible with a Physician's Professional Obligations?* Theor Med Bioeth. 2008; 29: 171-185.

272 MEANEY J, CASINI M, SPAGNOLO AG. *Objective Reason for Conscientious Objection in Health Care.* Natl Cathol Bioeth Q. 2012; 12 (4): 611-620, p. 613.

273 COMITATO NAZIONALE PER LA BIOETICA (CNB). *Conscientious Objection and Bioethics* (30 July 2012). Rome: Presidenza del Consiglio dei Ministri, Dipartimento per l'Informazione e l'Editoria; 2012 (accessed 11.11.2014, at: http://www.palazzochigi.it/bioetica/eng/pdf/Conscientious_objection_bioethics_12_06_2012.pdf).

274 WOLFF R. *Conscientious Objection: Time for Recognition as a Fundamental Human Right.* ASILS Int Law J. 1982; 6: 65-95, p. 82.

The right to conscientious objection has been upheld in Italy, for example, as a constitutional right even against what the modern Italian Constitution calls a "sacred duty", i.e. defending the Fatherland through military service.[275] The Italian Constitutional Court has accepted that the constitution grants the right to conscientious objection in the case of mandatory military service and to health care workers. They ruled that "there is no guarantee of inalienable rights and fundamental freedoms without a corresponding set of constitutional protections for that privileged and intimate relationship of a person with himself that is the cultural and spiritual basis and foundation of ethical-legal values".[276]

Ultimately, according to the court, "the individual conscience enjoys constitutional protection as an important constitutional principle that makes possible the reality of fundamental human freedoms belonging to the realm of the virtual expression of the inviolable rights of the individual in social life".[277] We are dealing with a general principle that enjoys constitutional protection in some countries and therefore can in no way be considered simply "an exception" to the law.

3.3.1.1. History and Present

Ancient texts from Greek literature, philosophy and dramaturgy, the philosophical writings of the Roman Stoics, and the Bible as cited earlier give us varied examples of this kind of witness by men and women. No in-depth discussion of conscience can be complete without making reference to the Greek masterpiece, Antigone. Sophocles in his tragedy has the protagonist disobey the unjust positive law promulgated by her uncle, the king, in order to obey the unwritten laws of the gods.[278] These laws are unchangeable and eternal; obeying them or not determines one's afterlife; Antigone senses that she would stand condemned in front of the gods, where she to obey the order of the king and fail to bury her brother. Her inner voice is following an absolute, moral command, which is precisely what a well-formed conscience should do. Aristotle would later refer to this literary example to draw the distinction between positive laws and the natural law.[279]

---

275 CASAVOLA FP. *L'Obiezione di Coscienza tra Libertà e Responsabilità* in LIVERANI PG (editor). L'Obiezione di Coscienza tra Libertà e Responsabilità. Siena: Cantagalli; 2013: 19-24, p. 22.276 ITALIAN
276 CONSTITUTIONAL COURT. *Sentenza N. 467* (16 December 1991). English Trans. MEANEY J. Rome; 1991 (accessed on 18.07.2011, at: http://www.cortecostituzionale.it/actionPronuncia.do).
277 *Ibid.*
278 SOPHOCLES. *Antigone; Oedipus the King; Electra.* English Trans. DAVY H, KITTO F. Oxford:Oxford University Press; 1994: Verses 453-457, p. 16-17.
279 ARISTOTLE. *Rhetorics.* 1373b, 1375ab.

What happens, when a fundamental law is broken, whether knowingly or not, is shown in Oedipus' case, for he is hounded by the Furies for having killed his father and married his mother. One needs to point out, of course, that the ethical understanding is not yet very developed in Sophocles' play, since personal responsibility seems irrelevant to the question of guilt and its punishment. The point is that a fundamental disorder has been brought into the world through Oedipus' parricide and his incestuous marriage with his mother. The gods, nay the cosmos itself, will not stand it; this explains the plague at the beginning of the play. That Oedipus as well as his parents had tried everything to avoid the fulfillment of the prophecy does not count in their favor. Oedipus is still haunted by the Furies.

Similarly, in the plays regarding Orestes, he (and in some versions also his sister Electra) is pursued by the Erinyes for killing his murderous mother, even though he was ordered to do so by Apollo.[280] When asked by Menelaus what illness is overcoming him, he replies at line 396 "sunesis" which many modern scholars have seen as echoing modern ideas of "conscience".[281] A sense of guilt seems to be strongly present in Ancient Greek culture, as well as the awareness that it is passed on through the generations. The Erinyes are, one could argue, a personified bad conscience, pursuing people until they are freed by the gods. The French philosopher, Simone Weil, even spoke of the "haunted conscience" of the Greeks, stemming from their destruction of Troy.[282]

From ancient to modern times conscience issues have been a subject of passionate societal debate. Already in the 16th century, England and Russia recognized conscientious objection to military service for certain groups.[283] Nevertheless, laws protecting conscientious objection were mainly passed in the 20th century. France waited until December 1963 to create a legal category of conscientious objector to military service.[284]

In the health care field, laws recognizing conscientious objection typically accompanied the depenalization or legalization of abortion.[285] This was the case in the majority of European nations and the US. The Charter of Fundamental Rights of the European Union from 2000 reaffirms this right recognized by the vast majority of its member states. "The right to conscientious objection is recognised, in accordance with the national laws governing the exercise of this right".[286] The Council of Europe has also recognized the importance of legal recognition for conscientious objection. "The right of conscientious objection is a

---

280 As Henry Chadwick points out, only with Euripides does the theme of conscience become prominent; he uses the term "to become aware of oneself", which means to be conscious of an inner conflict, for which the Greek term is *syneidesis*. CHADWICK H. Betrachtungen über das Gewissen..., p. 11.
281 WRIGHT M. *Euripides: Orestes*. London: Gerald Duckworth & Co. Ltd.; 2008: p. 56.
282 WEIL S. *Dieu dans Platon* in CAMUS A. (ed.). La Source Grecque. Paris: Gallimard; 19535: 67-126, p. 77.

fundamental aspect of the right to freedom of thought, conscience and religion enshrined in the Universal Declaration of Human Rights and the European Convention on Human Rights. Most Council of Europe member states have introduced the right of conscientious objection into their constitutions or legislation. There are only five member states where this right is not recognized".[287]

In 2011, so relatively recently, over 300,000 communications were received by the US Department of Health and Human Services, the vast majority in favor of retaining the strengthened conscience protections of President Bush, during the 60 day public comment period before the Barrack Obama administration could modify the George W. Bush administration Regulation for the Enforcement of US Federal Health Care Provider Conscience Protection Laws.[288] What constitutes an acceptable basis for conscientious objection by health care workers is controversial and therefore requires solid grounding in both ethics and legal theory. It is also important to recall that conscientious objection is the most important reality in health care worker conscience conflicts.

3.3.1.2. Academic Discussion Concerning Conscientious Objection

Within the academic literature a wide range of positions are taken.[289] Some think that "If people are not prepared to offer legally permitted, efficient, and beneficial care to a patient because it conflicts with their values, they should not be doctors".[290] This is, however, an extreme position that few bioethicists hold.

When the American College of Obstetricians and Gynecologists (ACOG) ethics committee issued an opinion in 2007 that ACOG members should be willing to violate their consciences if their convictions conflict with patient well-being, it ignited criticism of displaying "gross illogic and ideological bias".[291] The ACOG committee opinion is important because one of

283 SUADEAU J. L'Objection de Conscience ou le Devoir de Désobéir. Valence: Editions Peuple Libre; 2013: p. 56.

284 Ibid. p. 57.

285 For a comprehensive treatment of conscientious objection legislation relating to health care in Europe see: KUBALA MT. Obiezione di Coscienza e Rivendicazione Abortista in Europa [dissertation]. Rome: Pontifical University of the Holy Cross; 2013: p. 128-184.

286 EUROPEAN PARLIAMENT, COUNCIL AND COMMISSION. Charter of Fundamental Rights of the European Union (18 December 2000). Brussels; 2000: Art. 10 § 2. (accessed on 22.11.2014, at: http://www.europarl.europa.eu/charter/pdf/text_en.pdf).

287 PARLIAMENTARY ASSEMBLY OF THE COUNCIL OF EUROPE. *Recommendation 1518* (2001): *Exercise of the Right of Conscientious Objection to Military Service in Council of Europe Member States* (23 May 2001). Strasbourg; 2001 (accessed on 22.11.2014, at: http://www.refworld.org/docid/5107cf8f2.html).

288 UNITED STATES DEPARTMENT OF HEALTH AND HUMAN SERVICES (HHS). *Regulation for the Enforcement of Federal Health Care Provider Conscience Protection Laws* (23 February 2011). Washington DC; 2011(accessed on 11.11.2014, at: http://edocket.access.gpo.gov/2011/pdf/2011-3993.pdf).

the grounds for revocation of certification in female reproductive medicine in the US is violating ACOG or American Board of Obstetricians and Gynecologists (ABOG) rules or ethical principles.[292] Furthermore, this opinion has been re-affirmed in subsequent years. Princeton University's Professor Robert George pointed out how partisan and demagogically ideological this document is as a "power play" by pro-abortion zealots. "The greatest irony of the report is its stated worry about physicians allegedly imposing their beliefs on patients by, for example, declining to perform or refer for abortions-or at least declining to perform abortions or provide other services in emergency situations. The assumption here is the philosophical one that abortion, even elective abortion, is 'health care' and that deliberately killing babies in their mother's wombs is morally acceptable and even a woman's right. The truth is that the physician who refuses to perform abortions or the pharmacist who declines to dispense abortifacient drugs coerces no one. He or she simply refuses to participate in the destruction of a human life-the life of the child in utero".[293]

The broadly based criticisms and rejection of the ACOG committee opinion by doctors and ethicists helped to motivate the George W. Bush administration to strengthen enforcement procedures for existing federal conscience protection measures. As a matter of fact, this "opinion" did not become a firm policy with the potential to exclude obstetricians and gynecologists with consciences that prevent them from carrying out abortions or referring for them from being certified to practice medicine in their field. "Perhaps the most serious defect of the ACOG opinion is its failure to grasp, let alone to analyze, the nature, depth and the dimensions of the claim for protection of healthcare providers' rights of conscience. ACOG presents that merely as a claim for accommodation, based on principles of professional expediency".[294] Some of the opinions expressed by the ACOG committee are nonetheless valuable. "Finding a balance between respect for conscience and other important values is critical to the ethical practice of medicine".[295] It is, however, vital to understand the true relative importance of conscience and other rights as I discussed in chapter two.

---

289 DAVIS JK. *Conscientious Refusal and a Doctor's Rights to Quit.* J Med Philos. 2004; 29: 75-91; MAY T, AULISIO MP. *Personal Morality and Professional Obligations. Right of Conscience and Informed Consent. Perspect Biol Med* 2009; 52: 30-38.

290 SAVULESCU. Conscientious Objection…, p. 294.

291 BRUGGER EC. Abortion, Conscience, and Health Care Provider Rights (26 July 2012). Princeton; 2012 (accessed on 21.11.2014, at: http://www.thepublicdiscourse.com/2012/07/5902/).

292 ROUSSE ST. *Professional Autonomy in Medicine: Defending the Right of Conscience in Health Care Beyond the Right to Religious Freedom.* Linacre Q. 2012; 79 (2): 155-168, p. 160.

293 GEORGE. *Conscience and its Enemies,* p. 159.

294 WARDLE LD. *Rights of Conscience vs. Peer-Driven Medical Ethics: ACOG and Abortion* in KOTERSKI JW (editor). *Life and Learning XVIII: Proceedings of the Eighteenth University Faculty for Life Conference.* Bronx: University Faculty for Life; 2011: 23-56, p. 35.

295 AMERICAN COLLEGE OF OBSTETRICIANS AND GYNECOLOGISTS (ACOG) COMMITTEE ON ETHICS. *The Limits of Conscientious Refusal in Reproductive Medicine ACOG Committee Opinion no. 385.* Obstet Gynecol. 2007; 110: 1203-1208, p. 1205.

3.3.1.3. Autonomy

The academic discussion on conscientious objection is tied up with changing perceptions of the doctor-patient relationship. It has moved from the classical relationship based on the subjection and obedience of the patient to the physician for his own good, which often degenerated into "paternalism", to a relationship mainly based on the patient's autonomy. An exaggerated self-determination on the part of the patient, however, exposes the physician and other health care personnel to the risk of being transformed into mere technicians, the passive executors of the patient's will, which is not acceptable since they have their own moral autonomy.[296]

It logically follows, however, that if a patient's (or citizen's) self-determination is seen as a paramount value, the same protection must be granted for the freedom of conscience of the subject who is called upon to act. So, we are faced with a twofold requirement: on the one hand, to protect the physician's and health workers' autonomy according to their conscience; on the other hand to understand what the foundation of conscientious objection in the health-care professions field is.

"Behaving according to one's own science and one's own conscience" is the responsibility of members of the medical profession.[297] The consciences of health care workers are guided by codes of professional ethics. For example, the *Physician's Oath,* adopted by the 1948 General Assembly of the World Medical Association in Geneva, includes the words: "I will practice my profession with conscience and dignity".[298]

The 2014 Code of Medical Conduct of the Italian Medical Association chronologically places the rights of conscience before clinical principles in article 22: "The Physician who is requested to perform an intervention which is at odds with his conscience or with his clinical principles can refuse to participate in it unless that refusal causes serious and immediate injury to the patient's health and must also provide the citizen with all useful information and clarifications to allow the realization of these services".[299] We can observe that in this professional code of ethics conscience is given much more scope than is usually granted in court cases. It is a principle that can be applied to all professionals working in health care, medical doctors,

---

296 DAAR JF. *A Clash at the Bedside: Patient Autonomy v. A Physician's Professional Conscience.* Hastings Law J. 1993; 44: 1241-1289, p. 1247.

297 GAMBINO, SPAGNOLO. *Ethical and Juridical Foundations...*, p. 3.

298 WORLD MEDICAL ASSOCIATION (WMA). *Physician's Oath* (September 1948). Geneva; 1948 (accessed on 18.07.2011, at: http://www.mma.org.my/Portals/0/Declaration%20of%20Geneva.pdf).

299 FEDERAZIONE NAZIONALE DEGLI ORDINI DEI MEDICI CHIRURGHI E DEGLI ODONTOIATRI (FNOMCEO). *Codice di Deontologia Medica* (18 May 2014). English Trans. MEANEY J. Rome; 2014 (accessed on 22.11.2014, at: http://www.fnomceo.it/fnomceo/Codice+di+Deontologia+Medica+2014. html?t=a&id=115184).

nurses, midwives, pharmacists, etc. and which has never been seen as contrary to the law. This reflects the fact that health care continues to be based not on mere bureaucratic tasks, but on the personal responsibility of health professionals. This implies the need for health professionals not to be forced to carry out an intervention that they feel is unjust. They need to be able to act in a manner consistent with both their own assessment of what is medically relevant in each concrete case, and respect for their moral conscience.

An optimal doctor/patient relationship must include respect for the conscience and values of each of the parties. In fact, respect for conscience rights is an indispensable condition for the creation of a close doctor/patient relationship that is not merely a bureaucratic or contractual relationship.[300] It is frequently understood, however, that limits can be placed on the rights of conscience if a threat of serious and immediate injury to the patient's health exists.

3.3.2 The Legal Basis for Conscientious Objection

The ideological conflict over abortion has enflamed conscience problems in the health care arena. Conscientious objection was not a common practice in medicine internationally until the latter half of the 20th century when abortion was increasingly legalized and new technologies like in vitro fertilization were developed.[301] In many countries, including the US at both the federal and state level, laws explicitly endorsing the right to conscientious objection of medical personnel were passed in the wake of abortion legalization.[302] In some countries like Italy, the vast majority of doctors officially declare themselves to be conscientious objectors raising fears that access to abortion could be compromised.[303] The unfortunate end result is that rights of conscience for health care professionals have become closely linked to reproductive health laws and politics with some tendency to accept or reject conscience rights solely on the basis of one's position against or in favor of legalized abortion.[304] This is highly problematic, since conscience rights in medicine go far beyond the abortion issue, and the goal of providing easier access to any given procedure should never determine which human rights are upheld or not.

---

300 BURKE BJ. *The Loss of a Physician's Freedom of Conscience Will Result in the Breakdown of Patient Autonomy within the Doctor-Patient Relationship*. Linacre Q. 2009; 76 (4): 417-426, p. 424.

301 TURCHI V. *Nuove forme di obiezione di coscienza*. Stato, Chiese e pluralismo confessionale (October 2010). Milan; 2010 (accessed on 18.11.2014, at: http://www.statoechiese.it/images/stories/2010.10/turchi_nuove.pdf)

302 GOLD A. *Physicians' "Right of Conscience"-Beyond Politics*. J Law Med Ethics. 2010; 38 (1): 134- 142, p. 134.

303 PAVONE G. *Medici Obiettori: Un Problema Italiano*. La Repubblica (17 November 2011). Rome; 2011 (accessed on 08.10.2014, at: http: //d.repubblica.it/argomenti/2011/11/17/news/medici_obiettori- 668839/)

304 GOLD. *Physicians'...*, p. 139.

Resolution 1763 of the Parliamentary Assembly of the Council of Europe entitled "The Right to Conscientious Objection in Lawful Medical Care" from 7 October 2010 provides a concrete legislative approach that is respectful of conscience rights. The resolution explicitly guarantees the right of conscientious objection for both individual and institutional health care providers when taking a human life is legal. "No person, hospital or institution shall be coerced, held liable or discriminated against in any manner because of a refusal to perform, accommodate, assist or submit to an abortion, the performance of a human miscarriage, or euthanasia or any act which could cause the death of a human foetus or embryo, for any reason".[305]

British MP Christine McCafferty began the process that ended with the Council of Europe's resolution with a report entitled *Women's Access to Lawful Medical Care: The Problem of the Unregulated Use of Conscientious Objection*. The report took a position strongly in favor of limiting conscientious objection and explicitly denied the existence of a right to conscientious objection for institutions.[306] "According to international human rights law, the right to freedom of thought, conscience and religion is an individual right and, therefore, institutions such as hospitals cannot claim this right".[307] The Council of Europe's Parliamentary Assembly Committee on Equal Opportunities for Women and Men endorsed the "McCafferty Report" and actually proposed amendments further limiting the right to conscientious objection to "ensure that national healthcare systems require that healthcare providers receive training on how to perform all legal reproductive health services, irrespective of whether the student or trainee objects to performing them, in order to ensure access to healthcare services in emergency and other situations in which conscientious objection is not applicable".[308]

In the end, the Parliamentary Assembly of the Council of Europe, through the use of amendments, completely reversed the thrust of McCafferty's draft resolution so that it became a re-affirmation of the right of conscientious objection in the health care field for individuals

303 PAVONE G. *Medici Obiettori: Un Problema Italiano*. La Repubblica (17 November 2011). Rome; 2011 (accessed on 08.10.2014, at: http: //d.repubblica.it/argomenti/2011/11/17/news/medici_obiettori- 668839/)
304 GOLD. *Physicians'...*, p. 139.
305 PARLIAMENTARY ASSEMBLY OF THE COUNCIL OF EUROPE. *Resolution 1763 The Right to Conscientious Objection in Lawful Medical Care* (7 October 2010). Strasbourg; 2010 (accessed on 19.11.2014, at: http://assembly.coe.int/Mainf.asp?link=/Documents/AdoptedText/ta10/ERES1763.htm).
306 MCCAFFERTY C. *Women's Access to Lawful Medical Care: The Problem of the Unregulated Use of Conscientious Objection* (10 July 2010) Strasbourg; 2010 (accessed on 19.11.2014, at: http://assembly.coe. int/ASP/Doc/XrefViewPDF.asp?FileID=12506&Language=EN).
307 *Ibid.* p. 8
308 PARLIAMENTARY ASSEMBLY OF THE COUNCIL OF EUROPE COMMITTEE ON EQUAL OPPORTUNITIES FOR WOMEN AND MEN. *Committee Opinion Doc. 12389* (6 October 2010) Strasbourg; 2010 (accessed on 18.07.2011, at: http://assembly.coe.int/Main.asp?link=/Documents/WorkingDocs/ Doc10/EDOC12389.htm).

and institutions. The central problem that the parliamentarians attempted to resolve in practice was balancing the right of conscientious objection in the health care field with the right of persons to access lawful medical interventions. They did not, however, provide a theoretical basis for their decision.

The Swedish delegation was against the Council of Europe resolution. Their national parliament went so far as to vote on 11 May 2011 to approve a foreign affairs committee report vowing to work internationally against the 2010 resolution by the Parliamentary Assembly of the Council of Europe in favor of conscience rights in the health care field.[309] Sweden, in fact, is an isolated example.[310] It is one of the very few countries that make no provision for the conscience rights of health care personnel and has had its policies challenged nationally and before the Council of Europe.[311] In practice, most medical personnel must be prepared to carry out any legal procedure which they are ordered to perform or face legal sanctions and in short order dismissal from employment or even employability in the medical field if they refuse in conscience to participate. The right to professional conscientious objection is denied to medical workers by the Swedish State in a manner more reminiscent of authoritarian regimes than of democratic human rights respecting states and has resulted in an official complaint being filed at the Council of Europe's European Committee of Social Rights.[312]

Such harsh measures are hard to explain when taken by liberal democracies or groups who self-identify as protectors of an ever-expansive number of personal liberties and rights. Forcing medical personnel to violate their deeply held beliefs contradicts the cherished liberal principle that everyone should be free to think and act as they wish with only minimal restrictions on what they can or cannot do. The O'Neill Institute for National and Global Health Law at Georgetown University and Women's Link Worldwide recently published a document entitled "Conscientious Objection and Abortion: A Global Perspective on the Colombian Experience" and held a joint event at Georgetown University on 27 October 2014 with two panel discussions to "explore comparative global analyses on reproductive rights and conscientious objection".[313]

---

309 SWEDISH PARLIAMENT. *Freedom of Conscience in Health Care* (11 May 2011). Stockholm; 2011 (accessed on 19.11.2014, at: http:// www.consciencelaws.org/background/society/society004.aspx).

310 Only Finland, Bulgaria and the Czech Republic among EU countries have similar policies denying the right to conscientious objection. HEINO A, GISSLER M, APTER D, ET AL. *Conscientious Objection and Induced Abortion in Europe*. Eur J Contracept Reprod Health Care. 2013; 18: 231-233, p. 232.

311 KISKA R. *Sweden's Aggressive Attack on Conscience Challenged Before the Council of Europe*. Zenit (14 June 2014). Rome; 2014 (accessed on 19.11.2014, at: http: //www.zenit.org/en/articles/sweden-saggressive-attack-on-conscience-challenged-before-the-council-of-europe).

312 *Ibid.*

313 WOMEN'S LINK WORLDWIDE. *Balancing Conscience and Women's Reproductive Rights* (24 October 2014). Madrid; 2014 (accessed 18.11.2014, at: http://www.womenslinkworldwide.org/wlw/new.php?modo=detalle_prensa&dc=469).

Persons attending the event reported speakers equating conscientious objection with "torture" and "war crimes" and even suggesting that instead of the term "conscientious objection" the phrase "arbitrary refusal to care" or "refusal of services" should be used in an attempt to erode support for conscience protections.[314] This is part of a concerted international effort to reverse laws and policies that recognize conscience rights in health care.

The legalization of abortion in many countries in the last few decades as well as recent laws permitting euthanasia and also technological developments, such as the generation of human embryos in a laboratory context, have led to a multiplication of circumstances where medical professionals who refuse to participate in the killing of human beings feel obliged to invoke the right to conscientious objection. These medical professionals point out that several relatively recently legalized procedures violate both the Hippocratic Oath and traditional codes of conduct for the medical profession thereby causing conflicts of conscience.[315] Professor Marc Wicclair notes that literature searches failed to find examples of medical practitioners as conscientious objectors before the 20th century.[316]

New technologies both allow greater interventions impacting human lives, from conception to the end phases of life, and raise a growing number of relevant ethical questions for the consciences of health care personnel.[317] Physicians and other health care workers, in fact, are frequently called upon to perform biomedical interventions that, even when normatively legitimated, are unacceptable from the perspective of many individuals' moral consciences.[318] This is especially acute in the field of medicine where it is generally accepted that respect for human life and non maleficence are core values of the profession.[319]

The medical conscientious objection debate has become a focal point of legislation, court decisions and media attention. Even when laws explicitly provide for the right to conscientious objection, this right is periodically the object of controversy with regards to its application.

---

314 PARLIAMENTARY NETWORK FOR CRITICAL ISSUES. *Georgetown Law Entity Co-Authors Document Targeting Conscientious Objection.* Parliamentary Network E-News. 2014; 8 (10): November 2014 (accessed on 29.11.2014, at: http://www.pncius.org/index.aspx).

315 "Imagine: being declared persona non grata in medicine merely for wishing to abide by an ethic that was considered mandatory for all doctors as recently as forty years ago". SMITH J. Protecting the Careers of Medical Professionals Who Believe in the Hippocratic Oath (27 May 2009). Powell River; 2009 (accessed on 12.11.2014, at: http://www.consciencelaws.org/issues-legal/legal048.html).

316 WICCLAIR MR. *Conscientious Objection in Health Care an Ethical Analysis.* Cambridge: Cambridge University Press; 2011: p. 14.

317 TURCHI. *Nuove Forme...*, (accessed on 25.10.2014, at: http://www.statoechiese.it/images/stories/2010.10/turchi_nuove.pdf).

318 This was borne out by my empirical study of doctors. See Chapter 5.

319 BENN P. *Conscience and Health Care Ethics* in ASHCROFT RE ET AL (editors). *Principles of Health Care Ethics.* Hoboken: John Wiley& Sons, Ltd; 20072: 345-350.

In Italy Law n° 194 from 1978 legalized abortion, but article nine of that law recognizes that health care workers have the right to conscientious objection, even if there is disagreement concerning the exact extent of this right and exactly who benefits from it.[320]

In recent years, the use of birth control pills meant to be taken within 72 hours of unprotected sexual intercourse when it is feared an undesired pregnancy might occur and commonly known as the "morning-after pill" or "Emergency Contraception" has raised problems of conscience for both health care workers and institutions around the world.[321]

The principle reason some physicians have refused to write prescriptions for "Emergency Contraception" and many pharmacists have chosen not to dispense prescriptions for this drug is the belief that one of its main modes of operation is to prevent the implantation in the uterus of a human embryo.[322] This situation has led to legislation recognizing that other health professionals have the same rights to conscientious objection that physicians have exercised for some time in many countries. Some critics believe that these new laws have granted pharmacists and other professionals too much latitude and that this threatens patient health.[323] The Italian National Bioethics Committee, on the other hand, maintained that "medical doctors should have the right to recourse to conscientious objection in the case of prescribing the "morning-after pill".[324] I discuss this issue further in chapter four.

320 An examination of different cases with interpretative answers can be found in DI PIETRO ML, CASINI C, CASINI M. *Obiezione di Coscienza in Sanità. Vademecum.* Siena: Cantagalli; 2009.

321 CANTOR, BAUM. *The Limits of Conscientious…*, 2008-2012; BRAMSTED K. *When Pharmacists Refuse to Dispense Prescriptions.* Lancet. 2006; 367: 1219-1220.

322 This is a controversial claim, but there is scientific reasoning to support it. DI PIETRO ML, CASINI M, FIORI A, ET AL. *Norlevo e Obiezione di Coscienza. Medicina e Morale.* 2003; 53 (3): 411–455, p. 424- 432. A discussion of the divergent studies and views on the abortifacient or not potential of morning-after pills is included in this article. BELLUCK P. *Abortion Qualms on Morning-After Pill May Be Unfounded.* New York Times (5 June 2012). New York; 2012 (Accessed on 25.11.2014, at; http://www.nytimes.com/2012/06/06/health/research/morning-after-pills-dont-block-implantation-sciencesuggests.html?pagewanted=all&_r=0).

323 GRADY A. *Legal Protection for Conscientious Objection by Health Professionals.* Virtual Mentor. 2006; 8 (5): 327-331, p. 327. 324 COMITATO NAZIONALE PER LA BIOETICA. *Nota sulla Contraccezione D'Emergenza* (28 May 2004). Rome; 2004 (Accessed on 18.07.2011, at; http://www.palazzochigi.it/bioetica/testi/contraccezione_emergenza.pdf); *Id.Nota in Merito alla Obiezione di Coscienza del Farmacista alla Vendita di Contraccettivi di Emergenza* (25 February 2011). Rome; 2011 (Accessed on 18.07.2011, at; http://www.governo.it/bioetica/ pareri_abstract/Obiezione_coscienza20110225.pdf).

3.3.2.1. Protection for Conscientious Objection in Constitutions and Laws

As an interesting example, the exact phrase, "freedom of conscience", is not listed among guaranteed freedoms in the Italian Constitution, but the Italian constitutional Court has found that it is implicitly there, especially in article two which recognizes and guarantees "inviolable human rights".[325] Other articles with relevance to the right to conscientious objection are numbers 19 and 20 that cover freedom of religion and equal treatment and article 21 that guarantees freedom of expression and thought.[326] So, it is clear that conscientious objection rights may exist in constitutions without being explicitly included in the text.

Constitutional courts usually uphold this right in their rulings, if it is not written into the constitution, by extrapolating it from the right to freedom of conscience and religion. In this context, the Spanish Constitutional Court has ruled that conscientious objection is part of the contents of the fundamental right to ideological and religious freedom recognized by article 16.1 of Spain's constitution.[327] Other sentences from the same court, however, have not fully confirmed this opinion. In Spain, the 2011 revision of the Medical Deontological Code places new restrictions on conscientious objection, especially with regards to abortion, which will probably lead to legal challenges by medical doctors.[328]

Many countries with post-World War II constitutions in fact grant conscience rights and constitutional protection. The German Constitution recognizes conscience rights in article four on Freedom of Faith, of Conscience and of Creed. "(1) Freedom of faith and of conscience, and freedom of creed religious or ideological, are inviolable. (2) The undisturbed practice of religion is guaranteed. (3) No one may be compelled against his conscience to render war service as an armed combatant".[329] These articles of the German Constitution have been interpreted by the Federal Constitutional Court as guaranteeing the rights of those who refuse to perform military service or refuse to participate in performing abortions for reasons of conscience.

---

325 ITALIAN CONSTITUTIONAL COURT. *Sentenza N. 467...*, (accessed on 18.07.2011, at: http://www. cortecostituzionale.it/actionPronuncia.do).

326 ITALIAN REPUBLIC. *Constitution of the Republic of Italy* (22 December 1947). Rome; 1947 (accessed on 21.11.2014, at: https://www.senato.it/documenti/repository/istituzione/costituzione_inglese.pdf).

327 MARTIN DE AGAR JT. *Problemas Jurídicos de la Objeción de Conciencia. Scripta Theologica.* 1995; 2: 519-543.

328 RICO B. *Los Médicos Emprenden Acciones Contra el Nuevo Código Ético Profesional. Granada Hoy* (3July 2011). Granada; 2011 (accessed on 18.07.2011, at: http://www.granadahoy.com/article/granada/1012493/ los/medicos/emprenden/acciones/contra/nuevo/codig o/etico/profesional.html).

329 PARLIAMENTARY COUNCIL OF THE FEDERAL REPUBLIC OF GERMANY. *Basic Law for the Federal Republic of Germany.* Berlin: Federal Law Gazette; 1990: (accessed on 18.07.2011, at: http://www. constitution.org/cons/germany.txt).

Other nations have included conscience clauses in laws, particularly those permitting abortion. In Israel their 1977 Interruption of Pregnancy Law states: "Where approval under this Law has been given, a gynaecologist shall not for this reason be required to interrupt the pregnancy if such is contrary to his conscience or medical judgment".[330] Austria's Federal Law 60 of 23 January 1974 states that: "No one may be in any way disadvantaged because he or she has performed a justified abortion, or taken part in it, or because he or she has refused to perform or take part in such an abortion".[331]

As a general rule, the right to freedom of conscience is recognized by law at the national, European and international levels. The best known examples are article 18 of the 1948 Universal Declaration of Human Rights and article 18 of the 1966 International Convenant on Civil and Political Rights. The latter states unequivocally that "Everyone shall have the right to freedom of thought, conscience and religion."[332] Article nine of the 1950 Convention for the Protection of Human Rights and Fundamental Freedoms and even the 2004 draft European Constitution in article II-70 dedicated to fundamental rights, recognize freedom of conscience.

Within discussions of human rights, conscientious objection is often linked to freedom of religion and freedom of conscience.[333] It is significant, however, that in the European Convention on Human Rights and Biomedicine of 4 April 1997, a clause on conscientious objection was pointedly not inserted. During the debate of the Parliamentary Assembly of the Council of Europe, an amendment inserting the right of conscientious objection was proposed, but then rejected. The parliamentary speaker expressed disapproval for including conscientious objection in the document since it is already present in several other conventions. As the literature in the field demonstrates, it is necessary to broaden the reasons that form the basis for conscientious objection as well as the underlying ethical, philosophical, ideological and political principles for it.[334]

---

330 KNESSET OF THE STATE OF ISRAEL. *Criminal Law Amendment (Interruption of Pregnancy) Law.* Jerusalem: Knesset; 1977: (accessed on 18.07.2011, at: http://www.hsph.harvard.edu/population/abortion/ISRAEL.abo.htm).

331 AUSTRIAN PARLIAMENT. *Federal Law No. 60 of 23* January 1974. Vienna: Federal Law Gazette; 1974: (accessed on 18.07.2011, at: http://www.hsph.harvard.edu/population/abortion/Austria.abo.htm).

332 UNITED NATIONS GENERAL ASSEMBLY. *International Covenant on Civil…,* (accessed on 18.07.2011, at: http://www.ohchr.org/EN/ ProfessionalInterest/Pages/CCPR.aspx).

333 CHRISTIAN MEDICAL FELLOWSHIP UK. File 39: *The Doctor's Conscience.* London; 2009 (accessed on 24.08.2013, at: http://www.cmf.org.uk/publications/content.asp?context=article&id=25406).

334 TURCHI V. *I Nuovi Volti di Antigone. Le Obiezioni di Coscienza nell'Esperienza Giuridica Contemporanea.* Naples: ESI; 2009; D'AGOSTINO F. L'Obiezione di Coscienza Come Diritto. Iustitia 2009; 62: 177-182; VIOLA F. L'Obiezione di Coscienza Come Diritto. Persona y Derecho. 2009; 61: 53-71.

3.3.2.2. The Principle of Autonomy

There are several presuppositions in terms of the legal recognition of conscientious objection: a) the existence of a rule imposing requirements b) the existence of a second rule that, under certain specific formal conditions, allows someone not to fulfill the obligation created by the first rule. As a result, some laws provide for the possibility of invoking conscientious objection if a health care professional is required to comply with an obligation under the law but believes in conscience it is unjust and therefore goes against a norm that is considered more binding than obeying the legislation.

Certainly one could argue that every health worker has a subjective idea of what is right and what is unjust and that this could lead to chaos in the health care professions. The response to this assertion, however, is that the legal system does not respect/tolerate any and all opinions regarding the injustice of or ethical problems relating to a legal obligation. In fact, conscientious objection against the requirement to perform an action is legally recognized only when the moral sense of the individual deserves special consideration.

What therefore should be the criterion for judging whether a certain ethical judgment is or is not worthy of being accommodated? What would justify the adoption of a standard that allows disobedience to another law? Posing these questions helps us to understand why the legal basis for conscientious objection cannot be, or at least cannot only be, the rights to ethical and/or religious freedom as is frequently affirmed.

One should add another element. It is necessary that the "disobedience" to the law is motivated with reference to an objectively important basic value which is recognized by others and not just the individual who intends to invoke conscientious objection. What's more, this value must also be recognized as fundamental to the legislation that creates the obligatory standard.

Generally speaking, the legal system has no special regard for the private opinions of individuals and requires them to obey laws even when they consider them unjust. The reason behind binding everyone to obey the laws (*principle of legality*) is easily explained by the need to ensure the orderly and peaceful coexistence of society. All persons are required to contribute to the achievement of maintaining the common good through obeying the laws (principle of solidarity). In other words, ensuring the common good and the good of individuals is the organizing principle behind the law. This is the case despite the acknowledged possibility of poorly crafted laws or miscarriages of justice and a lack of unanimity regarding the justice of most laws.

The health care professions also have their own norms, which are there to specify the obligations of health professionals. As a consequence, if these norms are violated, the health care provider may be disciplined or criminally prosecuted. There are, however, some duties that the health professional is expected to carry out but which are not liable to criminal prosecution because they only relate to the code of professional ethics.

3.3.2.3. The Principle of Relevance

My position is that the recognition of the right to practice conscientious objection should not be interpreted simply as an expression of individual liberty — and thus a subjective right of autonomy. Conscientious objection in a country where basic human rights are recognized should be based upon principles closely tied to the very foundations of the legal system.[335] Otherwise, one runs the risk of nullifying the foundations that support the State and empty the principle of legality of its content. The right to conscientious objection, then, is only really reasonable if one discovers a link with the very purpose of the legal system.[336]

Since the mid-20th century, human rights charters, which are referenced by almost all recently adopted national constitutions, are principally concerned with the protection and promotion of human dignity. The first aspect of human dignity is respect for the value of existence and, in legal terms, the right to not be killed. The defense of human life is a foundational principle for both states and their legal systems. It is therefore logical that conscientious objection must be legally authorized at least in those cases where the individual's moral judgments pertain to respecting human life, the raison d'être of the State itself.

When the law moves away from the deep, structural reasons that govern modern legal systems, the protection of life and physical integrity, then it must acknowledge a genuine right to conscientious objection, not only as an individual freedom or right, but also as indicative of a collective value. In general, the legal system only allows for conscientious objection in certain well-defined areas. These have included military service, abortion, euthanasia and medically assisted procreation. A reason for this is because the law in these instances allows and organizes the killing of human beings as an immediate and certain effect of the actions of medical personnel (abortion and euthanasia) or as a possible eventuality (military service and medically assisted procreation). In this perspective, conscientious objection expresses unconditional faithfulness to some of the fundamental rights whose recognition is the source of law and for the protection of which the legal system exists, although it can make exceptions to this protection in some cases.[337]

---

335 Interestingly, Benn makes substantially the same argument from the perspective of medical codes of conduct. BENN. *Conscience and Health Care...*, p. 249-250.
336 DI PIETRO ML, CASINI C, CASINI M, SPAGNOLO AG. *Obiezione di Coscienza in Sanità. Nuove Problematiche per l'Etica e per il Diritto.* Siena: Cantagalli; 2005: p. 33-45.
337 EUSEBI L. *L'Obiezione di Coscienza del Professionista Sanitario* in RODOTA S, ZATTI P (editors). *Trattato di Biodiritto*, Vol. III *I Diritti in Medicina.* Milan: Giuffrè; 2011: 173-187, p. 173.

3.4 Conclusion

Conscientious subversion, civil disobedience and conscientious objection are all strategies for dealing with conflicts of conscience. As I have shown, the high degree of deception and illicit cooperation usually involved with conscientious subversion generally makes it an ethically unacceptable approach to use. It has the further drawback of undermining patient confidence in the honesty of health care professionals. There are some extreme circumstances where conscientious subversion could be justified, however, if the authorities are tyrannical and the conscientious subverter acts without lying or directly cooperating with evil. Non-violent civil disobedience is also a tactic that requires extreme circumstances. There must be a very serious unjust law and no other practical means to revoke it to justify civil disobedience. Finally, conscientious objection is the ethically preferred response in health care settings when a procedure or required action violates a person's conscience. It combines the witness value to touch the consciences of others of civil disobedience with an ethically acceptable safeguarding of conscience as long as patients are not abandoned or unattended in emergency situations.

Conscientious objection basing itself on the right to life of human beings is so fundamental as to be part of the bedrock of law. Since defending human life as an overriding concern is often taken for granted rather than explicitly formulated, it is easy for those opposed to conscientious objection to simply ignore it in their arguments. It is therefore important to re-affirm that doctors and health care professionals who invoke conscientious objection, in virtue of the objective foundation (principle of relevance) of their opposition are also defending justice and the common good.

To deny or severely limit health care workers' right to conscientious objection would be a serious ethical impoverishment of the medical profession and could send the message that ethics is not important.[338] It would also reduce physicians and others to being the mere executors of the will of others, creating a serious violation of human rights. Universal human rights are based on the principle of the equal dignity of every human being whether born or unborn, young or old, healthy or sick. Defending conscientious objection in the health care field affirms the principle of equality or nondiscrimination. Conscientious objectors affirm a noble principle "veritas non auctoritas facit ius" ("truth and not authority creates the law"), thereby reversing Hobbes' dictum.

---

338 GERRARD JW. *Is it Ethical for a General Practitioner to Claim a Conscientious Objection When Asked to Refer for Abortion?*. J Med Ethics. 2009; 35: 599-602; WICCLAIR. Is Conscientious Objection Incompatible…, p. 170-172.

CHAPTER 4:

CONSCIENCE RIGHTS FOR DIFFERENT CATEGORIES OF HEALTH CARE WORKERS

The topic of conscience rights and conflicts in health care is very much dominated by discussions focusing on medical doctors. In the preceding chapters and in chapter five, I have also focused on physicians. One reason for this is that general principles regarding conscience issues for health care providers obviously remain the same for all. Unique circumstances, nevertheless, arise for other categories of medical workers because of their different roles and status in the delivery of health care. The subordination of certain health care workers to medical doctors also puts them at greater risk of not having their conscience rights recognized and protected as effectively as those of physicians. Pharmacists, in particular, have been embroiled in much controversy concerning protecting their conscience rights in the face of the ethical challenges posed by the "morning-after pill". Therefore, it is important to discuss the conscience conflict situations and circumstances that arise for nurses and midwives, pharmacists and the current controversies surrounding "institutional conscience". In general, this discussion will concern "mid-level health workers" who generally receive shorter training than physicians but are expected to perform some similar duties and usually follow certified training courses and receive professional accreditation.[339]

Some arguments for conscientious objection imply that the conscience rights of doctors stem primarily from their high level professional status or practical benefits to the doctor/patient relationship that can come from accommodating the consciences of physicians.[340] It is interesting to note the possible negative consequences, such as "moral divestiture", of doctors stressed in the workplace by the moral distress of being forced to go against their consciences.[341] I am sympathetic to the argument that denying conscientious objection

339 LASSI ZS, COMETTO G, HUICHO L, ET AL. *Quality of Care Provided by Mid-Level Health Workers: Systematic Review and Meta-Analysis.* Bull World Health Organ. 2013; 91: 824-833. p. 24. [Online journal]. (accessed on 20.11.2014 at: http://www.who.int/bulletin/volumes/91/11/13-118786.pdf).
340 THOMASMA DC. *Beyond Medical Paternalism and Patient Autonomy: A Model of Physician Conscience for the Physician-Patient Relationship.* Ann Intern Med. 1983; 98 (2): 243-248; WHITE DB, BRODY B. *Would Accommodating Some Conscientious Objections by Physicians Promote Quality in Medical Care?.* JAMA. 2011; 305 (17): 1804-1805.
341 *Ibid.*

will have negative effects on the kind of persons entering and remaining in the medical profession.[342] If the right to conscientious objection of health care workers is based primarily on their high professional status, however, this leaves non-doctors at risk of being denied their conscience rights. What has happened with pharmacists in the area of conscientious objection is a clear example of this problem. I see conscientious objection as being justified mainly as a human right rather than as a professional prerogative, but it is also true that one characteristic of professionals is to be granted more freedom in their work than, for example, manual laborers. Therefore, I think it useful in this chapter to explore the professional status of nurses/midwives and pharmacists.

4.1 Nurses/Midwives

The practice of nursing is as ancient as health care delivery. According to the American Nurses Association, "Nursing is the protection, promotion, and optimization of health and abilities, prevention of illness and injury, alleviation of suffering through the diagnosis and treatment of human response, and advocacy in the care of individuals, families, communities, and populations".[343] Modern nurses have a specialized university education and are licensed by the state. They generally work as part of health care teams under the supervision of medical doctors.

Midwives are generally specialized nurses who care for women during pregnancy, labor, and the postpartum period, as well as caring for newborn infants. Their duties include taking measures aimed at preventing health problems in pregnancy, detecting abnormal conditions, procuring medical assistance when necessary, and the execution of emergency measures.[344] Because there are many serious ethical issues surrounding pregnancy, midwives are frequently at the forefront of conscience clashes faced by nurses. In fact, the oldest recorded conscience conflict involving medical workers was the resistance of the Hebrew midwives to the Egyptian ruler's decree to kill the newborn male children of the Hebrews.[345]

---

342 MEANEY J. *É un Bene per i Pazienti l'Obiezione di Coscienza del Medico?*. Medicina e Morale. 2011; 60 (5): 930-933, p. 931.

343 AMERICAN NURSES ASSOCIATION. *What is Nursing?* (accessed on 17.10.2014, at: http://www.nursingworld.org/EspeciallyForYou/What-is-Nursing).

344 WORLD HEALTH ORGANIZATION. *Health Topics: Midwifery*. (accessed on 19.11.2014, at: http://www.who.int/topics/midwifery/en/).

345 Exodus 1: 15-20.

4.1.1 Professional status

The professional status of nurses has evolved over time. In the latter half of the 19th century, with the creation of the first US schools of nursing following the "Nightingale plan", formal medical education for nurses began.[346] Nevertheless, nurses were expected to obey passively the orders of doctors, and if they disagreed with the decisions of a doctor played what has been called the "doctor-nurse game" in which nurses attempted to change a course of treatment by indirect means that allowed the physician to "save face".[347] Over time nurses have acquired ever greater medical responsibilities and training and recognized professional status.[348] Today the major nursing associations all assert the professional status of their members who are also licensed by the state.[349] This subordinate but professional status of nurses becomes a serious problem when the conscience of a nurse conflicts with those of an attending doctor. Fortunately, for US nurses over 80% of hospitals do not perform abortions, and all but four of the fifty US states have conscience clause laws.[350]

4.1.2 Deontological Codes

The American Nurses Association "Code of Ethics for Nurses With Interpretive Statements" that is currently in force states the following. "Where a particular treatment, intervention, activity, or practice is morally objectionable to the nurse, whether intrinsically so or because it is inappropriate for the specific patient, or where it may jeopardize both patients and nursing practice, the nurse is justified in refusing to participate on moral grounds".[351] This clearly supports the right of nurses to conscientious objection.

---

346 BENJAMIN M, CURTIS J. *Ethics in Nursing: Cases, Principles, and Reasoning.* Oxford: Oxford University Press; 2010: p. 96.

347 *Ibid.* p. 97.

348 As early as 1945, there was discussion of how to bring nursing to "professional maturity". KNIGHT BIXLER G, WHITE BIXLER R. *The Professional Status of Nursing.* Am J Nurs. 1945; 45 (9): 730-735, p. 730.

349 AMERICAN NURSES ASSOCIATION. *The Nonnegotiable Nature of the ANA Code for Nurses with Interpretive Statements* (8 December 1994). Silver Spring; 1994 (accessed on 22.11.2014, at: http://nursingworld. org/MainMenuCategories/Policy-Advocacy/PositionsandResolutions/ ANAPositionStatements/Position-Statements-Alphabetically/ prtetcode14446.html).

350 LATKOVIC MS. *Pro-Life Nurses and Cooperation in Abortion: Ordinary Care or Extraordinary Intervention?.* Natl Cathol Bioeth Q. 2004; 4 (1): 89-102, p. 94

351 AMERICAN NURSES ASSOCIATION. *Code of Ethics for Nurses With Interpretive Statements.* (15 November 2010). Silver Spring; 2010 (accessed on 22.11.2014, at: http://www.nursingworld.org/ MainMenuCategories/ EthicsStandards/CodeofEthicsforNurses/Code-of-Ethics.pdf).

There is an even stronger position statement by the US Association of Women's Health, Obstetric & Neonatal Nursing (AWHONN). "AWHONN supports the protection of an individual nurse's right to choose to participate in any reproductive health care service or research activity. Nurses have the right under federal law to refuse to assist in the performance of any health care procedure, in keeping with their personal moral, ethical or religious beliefs. The refusal should not jeopardize a nurse's employment, nor should nurses be subjected to harassment due to such a refusal".[352] This is a blanket statement of conscience rights in the field of reproductive health care, but it does accurately reflect the current protections under US Federal Law.

The Canadian Nurses Association is somewhat less supportive of conscientious objection since nurse are told they should "request" to be "accommodated" which is the language used for privileges not rights. "Ideally, the nurse would be able to anticipate practices and procedures that would create a conflict with his or her conscience (beliefs and values) in advance. In this case, the nurse should discuss with supervisors, employers or, when the nurse is self-employed, persons receiving care what types of care she or he finds contrary to his or her own beliefs and values (e.g., caring for individuals having an abortion, male circumcision, blood transfusion, organ transplantation) and request that his or her objections be accommodated, unless it is an emergency situation".[353] It is also unclear what kinds of "emergency situations" would be considered to override the consciences of Canadian Nurses.

The second part of article eight of the 2009 Italian Nurses' Deontological Code also touches on the conscience rights of nurses. "In the event of a persistent request for an action that goes against the ethical principles of the profession or personal values, nurses may avail themselves of the clause of conscience, to ensure the patient's safety and life".[354] This is a reference to the Italian Law which covers all health personnel and recognizes the right to conscientious objection with regard to abortion.

352 ASSOCIATION OF WOMEN'S HEALTH, OBSTETRIC & NEONATAL NURSING (AWHONN). *Ethical Decision Making in the Clinical Setting: Nurses' Rights and Responsibilities* (June 2009). Washington DC; 2009 (accessed on 22.11.2014, at: http://childrightsnurses.org/wpcontent/ uploads/2013/03/Resources_ Documents_pdf_ 5_ Ethics-copy1.pdf).
353 CANADIAN NURSES ASSOCIATION. *Code of Ethics for Registered Nurses*. Ottawa: CanadianNurses Association; 2008 p. 44 (accessed on 22.11.2014, at: https://cnaaiic. ca/~/media/cna/files/en/codeofethics. pdf).
354 COMITATO CENTRALE DELLA FEDERAZIONE & CONSIGILIO NAZIONALE DEI COLLEGI (IPASVI). *Codice Deontologico dell'Infermiere (2009)* Rome; 2009 (accessed on 12.11.2014, at: http://www. ipasvi.it/static/ english/the-nurses-deontological-code-2009.htm).

4.1.3 Legal cases

A 2013 verdict from an appeals court in Scotland was a victory for the right to conscientious objection. It was widely covered by newspapers and the BBC.[355] Two midwives, Concepta Wood and Mary Doogan, appealed a 2012 decision that recognized their right not to participate directly in abortions but refused to recognize a right to refuse administrative support for abortions.[356] Ultimately, however, they lost their case on appeal to the Supreme Court of the United Kingdom.

The two women were labor ward coordinators at the Glasgow Southern General Hospital and had long identified themselves as conscientious objectors to abortion. In 2007, the labor ward was also made responsible for an increasing number of abortions. They were subsequently ordered to supervise, support and delegate staff providing the abortion procedure. Both refused and, when the hospital refused to allow them not to cooperate with the scheduling and staffing of abortions, the midwives sued their hospital.

The first court ruled against Doogan and Wood, so they filed an appeal to the Scottish Court of Session claiming, among other arguments, a breach of Article 9 of the European Convention on Human Rights, which safeguards "freedom of thought, conscience and religion,"[357] on the grounds that requiring their participation in the process of providing abortions made them unacceptably morally complicit in it. The appellate judges ruled: "In our view it is not only the actual termination which is authorised by the Act for the purposes of section 4(1), but any part of the treatment which was given for that end purpose. Section 4(1) allows an individual to object to participating in "any" treatment under the Act. In our view the right of conscientious objection extends not only to the actual medical or surgical termination but to the whole process of treatment given for that purpose."[358] Thus, the April 2013 ruling of Doogan & Anor v NHS Greater Glasgow & Clyde Health Board, re-affirmed that the right of conscientious objection is a right that takes precedence over other rights/obligations in this case. This right of conscience bears a wide interpretation that extends beyond refusing direct participation in a procedure even to indirect administrative support of that procedure.

---

355 BBC NEWS. *Catholic Midwives Win Appeal over Abortion Case*. BBC News (24 April 2013). London; 2013 (accessed on 08.10.2014, at: http://www.bbc.com/news/uk-scotland-glasgow-west-22279857

356 OUTER HOUSE COURT OF SESSION. *Doogan & Anor v NHS Greater Glasgow & Clyde Health Board* (29 February 2012). Glasgow: ScotCS CSIH 32, appeal taken from Scot; 2012. p. 78-79. (accessed on 19.11.2014, at: http://www.scotcourts.gov.uk/opinions/2012CSOH32.html).

357 COUNCIL OF EUROPE. *European Convention on Human Rights* (4 November 1950). Rome: Council of Europe; 1950. Art. 9. (accessed on 19.11.2014, at: http://www.echr.coe.int/Documents/Convention_ENG.pdf

358 EXTRA DIVISION INNER HOUSE COURT OF SESSION. *Doogan & Anor v NHS Greater Glasgow& Clyde Health Board* (24 April 2013). Glasgow: ScotCS CSIH 36, appeal taken from Scot; 2013. p. 37. (accessed on 19.11.2014, at: http://www.bailii.org/scot/cases/ScotCS/2013/2013CSIH36.html).

Conscience rights are seen as ranking above hospital directives and even such competing rights as patient autonomy or access to medical procedures when the two conflict.

Unfortunately, the case was then appealed to the Supreme Court of the UK, which has only existed since 2009. Their decision came down on December 17, 2014. The judges decided to take a "strict constructionist" view of the 1967 Abortion Act as amended by the 1990 Human Fertilisation and Embryology Act. "It will immediately be apparent that the question in this case, and the only question, is the meaning of the words "to participate in any treatment authorised by this Act to which he has a conscientious objection".[359] They declared that scheduling abortions and most activities surrounding them, except for the actual procedure itself, cannot be legally protected by conscientious objection.

Doogan and Wood said "the ruling makes the conscience clause in practice meaningless for senior midwives in a labor ward."[360] The judges were aware that the conscientious objectors could have been accommodated relatively easily. The court pointedly refused to rule on the midwives' assertion that their rights under the European Convention on Human Rights, which explicitly guarantees the right to conscience, were violated. They passed this issue along to an employment tribunal case which is still pending.[361] Strange as it might seem, the UK Supreme Court will allow the lower court to rule whether the two midwives were victims of unjustified indirect discrimination on the ground of religion or belief under the UK Equality Act 2010.[362]

There have been many legal victories of nurses demanding that their conscience rights be respected. In the USA, Nurse Tony Lemly won a 2009 case appealed all the way to the Louisiana Supreme Court where she had refused to give out the morning-after pill and her hospital had punished her administratively.[363] In Canada, eight nurses challenged the policies of the Markham-Stoufville Hospital near Toronto to the Ontario Human Rights Commission. The commission ruled that staff with objections may not be required to participate in any way "in the administration, monitoring or documenting of the pregnancy termination process".[364]

---

359 SUPREME COURT OF THE UNITED KINGDOM. *Greater Glasgow Health Board (Appellant) v Doogan and another (Respondents) (Scotland)* (17 December 2014). London; 2014: §11 (accessed on 29.12.2014, at: https://www.supremecourt.uk/decided-cases/docs/UKSC_2013_0124_Judgment.pdf).
360 CATHOLIC NEWS AGENCY. *A 'Bullying' Move? UK Midwife Abortion Ruling Sparks Outcry* (19 December 2014). Los Angeles; 2014 (accessed on 29.12.2014, at: http://angelusnews.com/news/world/abullying-move-uk-midwife-abortion-ruling-sparks-outcry-7115/#.VKF78c8Dk).
361 SUPREME COURT OF THE UNITED KINGDOM. Greater Glasgow Health Board…, § 24.
362 Ibid.
363 ERTELT S. LA Nurse Wins State Supreme Court Battle in Plan B Conscience Case (20 May 2009). Lafayette; 2009 (accessed on 26.11.2014, at: http://www.louisianamedicalnews.com/la-nurse-wins-statesupreme- court-battle-in-plan-b-conscience-case-cms-1309).
364 CARELESS S. Nurses Triumphant! Human Rights Case Ends in Settlement: After a Difficult Five Year Struggle, Eight Ontario Health Care Professionals Win The Right to Choose (May 2009). Powell River; 2009 (accessed on 26.11.2014, at: http://www.consciencelaws.org/repression/repression007.aspx).

Twelve nurses won a legal case protesting against the University of Medicine and Dentistry of New Jersey that had changed its policy to require nurses to be present at and/or assist in abortion procedures.[365]

4.2 Pharmacists

Pharmacists are a category of health professionals whose conscience rights have generated much controversy in recent years. Exercising this health care specialty was not known for generating many ethical clashes for practitioners until the second half of the 20th century. The development and widespread use of new prescription drugs, such as the birth control pill, however, created new ethical problems for pharmacists. More recently, the increased dosages of the same drug to create "emergency contraception" or the "morning-after pill" meant to be taken within a few hours/days of sexual intercourse where the woman thinks she might conceive a child, created further ethical quandaries for some pharmacists. The RU-486 abortion pill and recent protocols for prescription drugs in view of physician assisted suicide have only added to the problems of conscience of many pharmacists.

Journalistic and even scholarly articles on the topic of conscientious objection by pharmacists frequently begin with extreme examples of persons whose prescriptions are not filled and the pharmacist refuses even to return the prescription to the person.[366] The authors of such articles are engaging in a transparent attempt to make conscientious objector pharmacists appear as moralizing and even intimidating or abusive zealots. Such extreme incidents are rare and furthermore do not accurately reflect the position of most ethicists who support conscience rights. For instance, Edmund Pellegrino affirms that health care providers do not have the right to impose their will on patients and should avoid moralizing and condemnatory statements when explaining why they cannot in conscience comply with a patient's request.[367] What such biased reporting on the pharmacist conscience rights issue fails to show is the terrible suffering of pharmacists who lose their jobs or face investigations by licensing agencies, go to court and are required to pay huge amounts like the $20,000 in costs Neil Noesen was assessed in Wisconsin for refusing to fill a birth control prescription.[368]

365 KORBE T. Court: New Jersey Nurses Don't Have to Assist With Abortions (23 December 2011). Washington DC; 2011 (accessed on 26.11.2014, at: http://hotair.com/archives/2011/12/23/court-newjersey-nurses-dont-have-to-assist-with-abortions/).

366 JONES C. *Druggists Refuse to Give Out Pill.* USA Today. (9 November 2004). Tyson's Corner; 2004 (accessed on 20.08.2014, at: http://usatoday30.usatoday.com/news/nation/2004-11-08-druggistspill_x.htm); COOPER WATT M. *Pharmacist Knows Best-Enacting Legislation in Oklahoma Prohibiting Pharmacists from Refusing to Provide Emergency Contraceptives.* Tulsa Law Rev. 2006; 42: 771-796, p. 771

367 PELLEGRINO ED. *La Conciencia del Medico, Cláusulas de Conciencia y Creencia Religiosa: una Perspectiva Católica.* Spanish Trans. SANTIAGO M. Cuadernos de Bioética 2014; 25 (3): 25-40, p. 39-40.

368 ANDERSON N. *Pharmacists with No Plan B: Freedom of Conscience and 'Reproductive Rights' Clash at the Local Drugstore.* Christianity Today, 1 August 2006; (accessed 20.08.2014, at: http://www.christianitytoday.com/ct/2006/ august/31.44.html?paging=off).

4.2.1 Professional status

Besides the challenges created by technological and legal changes is a much older conflict regarding the exact role of the pharmacist in delivering health care. Most pharmacists, and their professional associations, do not accept the viewpoint that sees medical doctors as those who should make all decisions and the pharmacist's role as restricted to the technical and passive preparing and filling of prescriptions.[369] In fact, John A. Gans, Executive Vice President and CEO of the American Pharmacists Association (APhA), responded negatively to the June 2005 resolution from the American Medical Association (AMA) annual meeting that in substance denigrated pharmacists' conscience rights and supported legislation requiring "individual pharmacists or pharmacy chains to fill legally valid prescriptions or to provide immediate referral to an appropriate alternative dispensing pharmacy without interference".[370]

It is quite understandable that pharmacists should be insulted when faced with the kind of contempt displayed by writers such as Wall and Brown who accept the view that pharmaceutical science is a typical example of "incomplete professionalization".[371] They affirm that pharmacists have "customers" while doctors have "patients" and use demeaning and extreme characterizations such as claiming that some conscientious objector pharmacists speak like Lewis Carroll's Humpty Dumpty.[372] Unsurprisingly, Watt and Brown and those who have similar beliefs are against recognizing any professional right of conscience for pharmacists.

It is important for a proper ethical consideration of the conscience issue for pharmacists and other health care workers to consider as objectively as possible the facts of the problem and not make emotional or red herring arguments as some opponents and even some supporters of conscience rights do. The issue really is what the conscience rights of pharmacists are.

---

369 CANTOR JD, BAUM K. *The Limits of Conscientious Objection-May Pharmacists Refuse to Fill Prescriptions for Emergency Contraception?*. N Engl J Med. 2004; 351: 2008-2012, pp. 2008-9.

370 GANS J. *Not Just a Matter of Conscience*. News Release, American Pharmaceutical Association (APhA), 23 June 2005; AMERICAN MEDICAL ASSOCIATION (AMA). H-120.947 *Preserving Patients' Ability to Have Legally Valid Prescriptions Filled* (18 June 2005) Chicago; 2005: p. 97. (accessed on 07.08.2014, at: http://www.ama-assn.org/ad-com/polfind/ Hlth-Ethics.pdf).

371 WALL LL, BROWN D. *Refusals by Pharmacists to Dispense Emergency Contraception: A Critique*. Obstet Gynecol 2006; 107: 1148-1151, p. 1148. 372 Ibid. p. 1149.

372 *Ibid*. p. 1149.

4.2.2 Deontological Codes

The official APhA policy adopted in 1998 upholds the conscience rights of pharmacists. "APhA recognizes the individual pharmacist's right to exercise conscientious refusal and supports the establishment of systems to ensure patients' access to legally prescribed therapy without compromising the pharmacist's right of conscientious refusal".[373] This policy was adopted at the national level in the United States and also at the state level by several member organizations of the APhA.[374] A poll of pharmacists by Pharmacy Times found that 62% of pharmacists agreed with the statement: "Pharmacists should be allowed to step away from dispensing the morning-after pill".[375]

Interestingly, the current code of ethics approved by the APhA includes a reaffirmation of the importance of conscience. "A pharmacist has a duty to tell the truth and to act with conviction of conscience".[376] At the same time, the Code of Ethics for Pharmacists acknowledges the problem of clashing moral and ethical approaches among health workers. "A pharmacist acknowledges that colleagues and other health professionals may differ in the beliefs and values they apply to the care of the patient".[377] Taken as a whole, this deontological code is quite supportive of pharmacists who refuse to compromise or violate their rights of conscience.

There is also a strong statement in heading III of the same code of ethics; "A pharmacist respects the autonomy and dignity of each patient".[378] Clearly, respecting the autonomy rights of patients should be a high priority for pharmacists. The reverse is also obviously true, i.e. patients should respect the autonomy and dignity of pharmacists, since we are dealing here with the general realm of human rights that apply to all human beings and not just specific categories of people.

In turn, the Italian Deontological Code for Pharmacists from 2007 states in article three that pharmacists "must work with full autonomy and professional consciousness in accordance with ethical principles, and always keeping in mind the patient's rights and respect for life".[379] This points in the direction of the need to legislate conscience protections when pharmacists must invoke conscientious objection to safeguard their ethical principles.

---

373 Cited in editorial by ECKEL F. *Pharmacist's Right to Choose?*. Pharmacy Times (1 July 2005). (accessed 06.08.2014, at: http://www.pharmacytimes.com/publications/issue/2005/2005-07/2005-07-9737).
374 BRAUER K. APhA *Delegates Passed a Conscience Clause for Pharmacists* (20 April 1999). (accessed on 06.08.2014, at: http://www.gargaro.com/pharmacy/).
375 ECKEL, *Pharmacist's Right*...p. 1.
376 AMERICAN PHARMACISTS ASSOCIATION (APhA). *Code of Ethics* (27 October 1994). Washington, D.C.; 1994 (accessed on 06.08.2014, at: http://www.pharmacist.com/code-ethics).
377 *Ibid.*
378 *Ibid.*
379 FEDERAZIONI ORDINI FARMACISTI ITALIANI (FOFI). *Codice Deontologico del Farmacista* (2007). English Trans. MEANEY J. Rome; 2007 (accessed on 21.10.2014, at: http://www.fofi.it/).

It is true that pharmacists were frequently not included in conscience protection legislation when the majority of these laws were created, but the explanation for these lacunae is chiefly that the laws were generally created in response to the liberalization of abortion, and pharmacists did not have anything to do with abortion at the time. In Italy, lawmakers were farsighted enough to include all health care personnel in article 9 of Law 194 of 1978 that recognized the right of conscientious objection to the practice of abortion.[380] In the United States the absence of laws protecting the rights of pharmacists was partially rectified at the state level when in the early 2000s pharmacists were required to fill prescriptions for the morning-after pill and many in conscience refused to do so. Bills protecting the conscience rights of pharmacists were introduced in 29 states.[381] State legislatures in Arizona, Arkansas, Georgia, Idaho, Mississippi, and South Dakota passed laws specifically protecting pharmacists who refused to cooperate in dispensing the morning-after pill, and Colorado, Florida, Maine, Illinois and Tennessee have broad medical conscience protection legislation that covers pharmacists.[382] One state, New Jersey, passed a radical law making it illegal for pharmacists to refuse to fill a prescription if their objection to doing so is for moral, religious or ethical reasons.[383] The greatest controversy in the press and legislatures came in 2005 and 2006 in the US but the issue of conscience conflicts for pharmacists has continued.[384]

4.2.3 Legal Cases

In the Pichon and Sajous v. France decision of 2 October 2001, the European Court of Human Rights in Strasbourg was unconvinced by the argumentation of French pharmacists who had refused to fill prescriptions for "morning-after pills".[385] The pharmacists appealed to the right to freedom of conscience and religion as laid down in article nine of the European Convention on Human Rights. At first, they were punished with a fine, even before the

---

380 ITALIAN PARLIAMENT. *Legge 22 maggio 1978, n. 194 Norme per la Tutela Sociale della Maternità e sull'Interruzione Volontaria della Gravidanza* (22 May 1978). art. 9. Rome; 1978 (accessed on 18.08.2014, at: http://www.salute. gov.it/imgs/C_17_normativa_845_allegato.pdf).

381 DUVALL M. *Pharmacy Conscience Clause Statutes: Constitutional Religious Accommodations or Unconstitutional Substantial Burdens on Women.* Am Univ Law Rev. 2005; 55: 1485-1521, p. 1488.

382 NATIONAL CONFERENCE OF STATE LEGISLATURES (NCSL) HEALTH PROGRAM. *Pharmacist Conscience Clauses: Laws and Information* (May 2012). Denver; 2012 (accessed on 20.08.2014, at: http://www.ncsl.org/research/health/pharmacist-conscience-clauses-laws-andinformation. aspx).

383 *Ibid.*

384 NATIONAL ASSOCIATION OF BOARDS OF PHARMACY (NABP). *Conscience Clause Controversy on Back Burner, but Still Simmering.* NABP Newsletter, 22 April 2011 (accessed on 20.08.2014, at: http://www.nabp.net/news/conscience-clause-controversy-on-back-burner-but-stillsimmering/).

385 LAMACKOVÁ A. *Conscientious Objection in Reproductive Health Care: Analysis of Pichon and Sajous v. France.* Eur J Health Law. 2008; 15 (1): 7-43.

definitive decision was reached, because they had not fulfilled their obligation to sell a drug prescribed by a medical doctor. The European Court of Human Rights argued that their invoking of the human right to freedom of conscience to justify conscientious objection in this case was groundless because article nine of the Convention does not always guarantee the right to conduct in the public domain that is dictated by a person's belief. They ruled that if the sale of a product is legal, pharmacists should not impose on others their beliefs. The judges added that pharmacists have many ways of expressing their beliefs outside the professional domain.[386] However, it is simply untrue that a pharmacist who declines to dispense abortifacient drugs coerces anyone.[387] Furthermore, coercing pharmacists to sell products that violate their consciences has been rightly condemned in other court rulings. A recognized private right to belief should come with safeguards not to be forced to perform an action seen in conscience as immoral.[388] The European Court of Human Rights failed to uphold properly human rights in the Pichon and Sajous v. France case.

Despite broad conscience protection in Illinois state law, Governor Rod Blagojevich, who was later impeached and jailed for corruption, signed an emergency rule valid for 150 days on 1 April 2005 forcing all pharmacists to dispense morning-after pills and creating a telephone hotline to report noncompliant pharmacists.[389] This was challenged in a court case, Morr-Fitz v. Quinn, as a violation of the Illinois Health Care Right of Conscience Act by several pharmacists. After 7 years, the Appellate Court of Illinois for the Fourth District ruled in 2012 that the State of Illinois could not force either pharmacists or pharmacies to dispense morning-after pills if it goes against their consciences.[390] In fact, the court was also applying an elementary legal principle. Just because the State does not forbid the sale of a drug, this does not automatically mean that all pharmacists are required to sell it.[391]

4.3 Institutions

Health care institutions are embroiled in the conscience issue as well as individual health professionals. Hospitals and other institutions have in fact received conscience

---

386 *Ibid.*

387 GEORGE. *Conscience and its Enemies…*, p. 159.

388 WOLFF. *Conscientious Objection…*, p. 82.

389 DUFRESNE B, MANAGAN N, MULLADY R. *Distribution of Birth Control by Pharmacists. The Vermont Legislative Research Shop*, 26 April 2005 (accessed on 18.08.2014, at: https://www.uvm.edu/~vlrs/Health/birthcontrolandpharmacists.pdf).

390 SAUNDERS W, SMITH M. *Pro-Life Pharmacists Win Huge Victory in Illinois Decision.* LifeNews.com, 24 September 2012 (accessed on 20.08.2014, at: http://www.lifenews.com/2012/09/24/prolife- pharmacists-win-huge-victory-in-illinois-decision/).

391 VISCHER. *Conscience and the Common Good…*, p. 165.

protections by US federal and state laws.[392] As mentioned earlier in the dissertation, the most important "conscience clause" legislation in the USA, the Church Amendment, came as a reaction to the Supreme Court's Roe v. Wade decision legalizing abortion, but the concrete case that motivated the law was one regarding institutional conscience. St. Vincent's Catholic hospital in Montana was ordered by a court to permit surgical sterilizations which their policies did not allow, and the US Congress reacted specifically to prevent this kind of legal coercion of health care institutions.[393] The paradigmatic case for most observers has been Catholic hospitals that refuse to permit the performance of abortions in their facilities, but other conscience cases arise as well. The conscience issues concerning health care institutions concern other realities as well, such as medical schools and pharmacies owned by individuals or institutions with conscientious objections to morning after pills.

4.3.1 Does Institutional Conscience Exist?

The first question that must be answered is at the heart of the scholarly debate on this issue. Can institutions have a "conscience"? Several academic authors, most notably Spencer Durland, Elizabeth Sepper and Bernard Dickens, have challenged the concept of institutional conscience and the legal protections that have been accorded to it.[394] These critics essentially claim that conscience is a faculty which only flesh and blood persons can possess. "Institutional conscience is fundamentally different from individual conscience but is mistakenly treated in legislation and academic discussion as equivalent. Legal fiction aside, a hospital is not a person; it is a physical structure within which providers give medical care. It does not perform procedures or counsel patients. It does not take lunch hours or vacations. And it does not have a conscience".[395]

On the opposite side of the institutional conscience debate are such scholars as Elliot Bedford, Grattan Brown and Daniel Sulmasy.[396] They all agree that institutions only have a conscience

---

392 For a timeline and summary of conscience rules in the United States since 1973 see AMERICAN ASSOCIATION OF PRO LIFE OBSTETRICIANS AND GYNECOLOGISTS (AAPLOG). *The Recent History of Conscience Rules* (26 July 2012). Eau Claire; 2012 (accessed on 24.10.2014, at: http://www.aaplog.org/physician-conscience-rights/the-recent-history-of-conscience-rules/).

393 CLARK BR. *When Free Exercise Exemptions Undermine Religious Liberty and the Liberty of Conscience: A Case Study of the Catholic Hospital Conflict.* Oregon Law Rev. 2013; 82 (3): 625-694, p. 644.

394 DURLAND S. *The Case against Institutional Conscience.* Notre Dame Law Rev. 2011; 86 (4): 1655- 1686; SEPPER E. *Taking Conscience Seriously.* Virginia Law Rev. 2012; 98: 1501-1575; DICKENS BM. *Conscientious Objection and Professionalism.* Expert Rev Obstet Gynecol. 2009; 4 (2): 97-100.

395 DURLAND. *The Case against...*, p. 1659.

396 BEDFORD EL. *The Concept of Institutional Conscience.* Natl Cathol Bioeth Q. 2012; 12 (3): 409-429; BROWN G. *Institutional Conscience and Catholic Health Care* in KOTERSKI JW (editor). *Life and Learning XVI: Proceedings of the Sixteenth University Faculty for Life Conference at Villanova University.* Washington, DC: University Faculty for Life; 2007: 413-422; SULMASY. What is Conscience..., p. 144.

by analogy to the conscience of individuals, so the criticisms of those opposed to recognizing institutional conscience are really a "straw man" argument. The real question is if the ethical principles or institutional conscience of groups merit protection or not. Nevertheless, Bedford in particular, makes a powerful case for institutional conscience being a meaningful reality. He introduces the concept of "social agency" as an aspect of human agency where an individual as a member of an institution acts in a responsible way on behalf of others.[397] This is a key point since a main criticism of institutional conscience is the assertion that hospitals or other institutions cannot possess the moral agency required for conscience. Bedford asserts that this moral agency exists in institutions through the social agency of its members authorized to act on behalf of the institution and make moral judgments.[398] Sulmasy sums up the defense of institutions having a conscience that can be safeguarded. "The conscience of an institution is rooted in the fact that it professes a set of fundamental moral commitments and it must act in accord with them".[399]

It is important to remember that the idea of institutional conscience having a substantial reality has been generally accepted in laws and practice. Thomas Nairn points out that an entire field of ethics, organizational ethics, exists to deal with circumstances when the values of an institution come into conflict either with internal or external controls.[400] Brown points out that hospitals do in fact require their employees to make judgments and act with reference to a common institutional mission.401 It is clear to all objective observers that institutions such as hospitals are not random aggregates of doctors, nurses, etc. and that the institution's identity and purpose is greater than the sum of its parts.[402] Hospitals and other institutions can be held legally responsible for failures in adhering to their own institutional guidelines, so it seems far-fetched to claim that these same institutions do not have ethical principles that can and should be recognized.

In a devastating critique, Bedford points out that the detractors of institutional conscience make self-contradictory arguments. Authors such as Sepper and Durland actually presuppose the validity of institutional conscience while arguing against its existence. They appeal to such manifestations of institutional conscience as decisions from the American College of Obstetricians and Gynecologists (ACOG), the American Medical Association (AMA) or even the US government to substantiate their case.[403] They can certainly claim that they disagree

---

397 BEDFORD EL. *The Act of Institutional Conscience: An Examination and Defense* [dissertation]. St. Louis: Saint Louis Univ.; 2014, p. 78.

398 *Ibid.* p. 80-81.

399 SULMASY. *What is Conscience...*, p. 143.

400 NAIRN TA. Institutional Conscience Revisited Catholic Institutions and Christian Ethics. New TheolRev. 2001; 14: 39-49, p. 46.

401 BROWN. *Institutional Conscience...*, p. 417.

402 SULMASY. *What is Conscience...*, p. 143.

403 BEDFORD. *Act of Institutional Conscience...*, p. 117.

with the institutional consciences of hospitals with prolife policies. But if they do so, then it is unreasonable to claim that these corporations do not have institutional consciences in the first place.

These academics appear to be motivated by an animus against the policies of Catholic and other hospitals that do not perform abortions rather than a true doubt about the existence of institutional conscience. In particular, they dislike The Ethical and Religious Directives for Catholic Health Care Services (ERDS) issued by the US Bishops Conference that govern the policies of Catholic hospitals in the USA and prohibit such procedures as abortions, sterilization and contraception.[404] Brieta Clark points out that in the USA, Catholic hospitals provide 20% of the acute care services and she sees this as "devastating" because in some communities the only hospital is religious and will not provide abortions or other procedures such as surgical sterilizations.[405] There is so much apprehension that Catholic hospitals are "taking over" health care in the USA by merging with other entities and thanks to the ERDS the merged hospital no longer permits abortions, etc. that an organization called Merger Watch was founded in 1996 to lobby against such mergers.[406] Groups are certainly free to criticize or protest the institutional consciences of Catholic corporations and others, but conscience rights remain and it is ethically and generally legally unacceptable to discriminate against the consciences of institutions and religious groups unless a procedure has been judged to be contrary to the goals of medicine or the common good by the vast majority of the profession.[407]

4.3.2 Conflicts Between Individual and Institutional Conscience

In recent years, new claims have been made against health care institutions stating that the positive claims of health care workers who feel obliged to offer such procedures as abortions should take precedence over institutional conscience rules prohibiting such actions. This is sometimes called "conscientious commitment".[408] As Professor Christopher Tollefsen points out, however, putting such a view into practice would effectively destroy

404 UNITED STATES CONFERENCE OF CATHOLIC BISHOPS. *Ethical and Religious Directives for Catholic Health Care Services* (17 November 2009). Washington DC; 20095 (accessed on 30.10.2014, at: http://www.usccb.org/issues-and-action/human-life-and-dignity/health-care/upload/Ethical-Religious-Directives-Catholic-Health-Care-Services-fifth-edition-2009.pdf).
405 CLARK. *When Free Exercise…*, p. 639-640.
406 MERGER WATCH. *In Medical Care, the Patients' Rights Must Come First*. New York; 2014 (accessed on 30.10.2014, at: http://www.mergerwatch.org/about/).
407 TOLLEFSEN CO. *Protecting Positive Claims of Conscience for Employees of Religious Institutions Threatens Religious Liberty*. Virtual Mentor. 2013; 15 (3) 236-239, p. 237.
408 DICKENS BM, COOK RJ. *Conscientious Commitment to Women's Health*. Int J Gynaecol Obstet. 2011; 113 (2): 163-166, p. 163.

some religious institutions. "Accordingly, I believe the idea of protections for positive rights of conscience for health care workers in Catholic (and many other religious) institutions, where the judgments of conscience in question run contrary to the foundational commitments of the institution, to be a non-starter: its facial deference to the rights of conscience actually conceals a deeper antipathy to the rights of conscience and religious liberty that are exercised not just by individuals acting in isolation from others, but by individuals acting cooperatively together with others to serve essential goods in accordance with their deepest religious and professional convictions.[409] Once again, institutional conscience is under attack from the perspective of individual conscience.

Clearly positive as well as negative rights of conscience exist. Wicclair points out correctly that positive conscience claims can merit protection for the same reasons that are valid for negative claims of conscience.[410] He concludes that negative conscience claims should not be selectively protected above positive claims. What Wicclair fails to address, however, is a fundamental difference between positive and negative rights. As I wrote in chapter two, negative rights tend to take precedence over positive ones because the latter are much more difficult to fulfill. It is apparent that guaranteeing a person's right not to be expelled from their homes is much more feasible, given the inherent scarcity of resources, than supplying a home to everyone that needs one. Positive claims of conscience also provide much greater challenges to the principle of legality. The consequences of allowing persons to act against laws positively as opposed to refraining from acting are more far reaching and difficult to manage.

The very delicate balance involved in negative conscientious objection could be overturned and would certainly be much more complicated if positive claims of conscience were added to the mix without careful deliberation. This helps to explain why, as even advocates of positive conscience admit, negative conscience claims "catalyzed the development of law, theory, and practice of conscientious objection in medicine".[411] It is a fact, lamented by some and approved by others, that typically only negative claims of conscience are protected by laws while conscience-based obligations to provide professionally permitted procedures or goods are not.[412] Furthermore, it is commonly admitted that the State can and should prevent individuals from acting on their conscientious judgments if protecting and promoting the common good requires it.[413]

---

409 TOLLEFSEN. *Protecting Positive Claims…*, p. 239.

410 WICCLAIR MR. *Negative and Positive Claims of Conscience*. Camb Q Healthc Ethics. 2009; 18: 14- 22, p. 16.

411 HARRIS LH. *Recognizing Conscience in Abortion Provision*. N Engl J Med. 2012; 367 (11): 981-983. p. 981.

412 WICCLAIR MR. *Conscientious Objection in Health Care: An Ethical Analysis*. Cambridge: Cambridge University Press; 2011: p. 230.

413 TOLLEFSEN CO. *An Absolute Liberty of Conscience?* (9 January 2009). Princeton; 2009 (accessed on 23.11.2014, at: http://www.thepublicdiscourse.com/2009/01/100/).

While freedom of conscience is not limited, conscientious objection may be circumscribed under some circumstances by both the State and institutions. "Were all conscientious objection claims equally reasonable, conscientious objection would be nothing more than a synonym for carte blanche permission to do whatever one wants irrespective of the rights of others".[414]

It remains a valid point, however, that the general category of positive conscience claims deserves to be considered and has not been adequately investigated by bioethicists.[415] The reasonable caveat to this, however, is that ethicists should recognize that appeals to positive conscience should rightfully pass a more strenuous test since accommodating them is generally much more onerous than negative ones. In the case mentioned above, health care workers exercising a positive right of conscience to perform non-permitted abortions, there are ample reasons why this should not be allowed. There is no overwhelming consensus that abortion fulfills the goals of health care. In fact, the opposite view was the norm until the last few decades and a substantial percentage of physicians, even a majority in many countries, do not see it as ethically permissible since it does not heal but instead takes a human life.[416] It is also clear that validating such a right of conscience would destroy such institutions as Catholic hospitals that would be forced to close down or commit civil disobedience rather than submit to the violation of their ethical stance against abortion.[417] This kind of severe violation of institutional conscience cannot be justified. Finally, the State could also not submit to such a positive right of conscience to commit abortion. If allowed, it would invalidate in practice any and all legal restrictions on abortion; gestational time limits, requiring certain conditions for abortion, etc. In effect, it would create a virtually unlimited right to abortion as long as doctors could be found willing to perform it.

414 VACCA MA. *A Reexamination of Conscience Protections in Healthcare*. Medicina e Morale. 2013; 62 (6): 1203-1207, p. 1205.
415 HARRIS. *Recognizing Conscience…*, p. 982.
416 HEANEY SJ. *Protecting Conscience in Health Care: Taking a Road Not Travelled*. Natl Cathol Bioeth Q. 2008; 8 (4): 673-680, p. 678.
417 Bishop Thomas Paprocki, a Chicago auxiliary bishop, stated that Catholic hospitals would have to shut down if the Freedom of Choice Act requiring abortion provision as a fundamental right passed in the USA. VEITH G. *Mandated Abortion Would Cause Catholic Hospitals to Close or Rebel* (11 March 2009). Denver; 2009 (accessed on 22.11.2014, at: http://www.patheos.com/blogs/ geneveith/2009/03/mandatedabortion-would-cause-catholic-hospitals-to-close-or-rebel/).

4.4 Conclusions

The foregoing discussion dealt with special cases of conscience rights in health care. I agree with the position of the Italian National Bioethics Committee that the exact professional status of health care workers is not what is most significant in determining their conscience rights. "The pharmacist as a citizen in a democratic society characterized by ethical pluralism, has the right not to perform an action, indicated under certain physiological conditions as scientifically capable of preventing the development of a human embryo, when it conflicts with their moral beliefs regarding the respect and protection due to a human being from the beginning of its development".[418] It is certainly true that the professional status of nurses, midwives and pharmacists has increased over time, but I believe that too much focus on "professional conscience rights" is misplaced. There is no ontological difference between doctors and nurses, and, as I showed in chapter two, this is a human rights issue not primarily a professional rights issue. Therefore, I do not see a compelling reason why a doctor should have more or less conscience rights than a pharmacist or other health care worker. What matters much more in justifying an appeal to conscience is the objective nature of the conflict of conscience.[419] In the health care field, a conscientious objection must also be rooted in fulfilling the goals of medicine.

Regarding the issue of institutional conscience, I am convinced by the arguments in favor of granting them conscience protections, under the same conditions as individuals. Although organizations do not have a personal conscience, they can and do have ethical guidelines which are a meaningful reality. Furthermore, as Bedford states, institutions have moral agency through the social agency of those who act on their behalf in making ethical decisions.[420] Arguments against the existence of institutional conscience seem to be motivated more by disagreement with some established ethical guidelines rather than a genuine belief that organizations cannot act conscientiously.

Finally, the recently formulated arguments that individual appeals to positive conscience claims should trump institutional conscience are problematic. Implementing positive rights in general requires more justification than negative ones since they clash more often with other rights and frequently have far reaching consequences. It is certainly true that positive conscientious obligations to act can be legitimate and deserve protection, but legal recognition for them must only be granted after careful consideration. In the specific case of a positive conscientious right to perform abortions, there are strong deontological, legal and practical reasons to reject this claim.

---

418 COMITATO NAZIONALE PER LA BIOETICA. *Note on the Pharmacist's Conscientious Objection to the Sale of Emergency Contraceptive Products* (25 February 2011). Rome; 2011 (accessed on 25.11.2014, at: http://www.governo.it/bioetica/eng/pdf/Pharmacist_conscientious_20110211.pdf).
419 MEANEY J, CASINI M, SPAGNOLO AG. *Objective Reason for Conscientious...*, p. 619.
420 BEDFORD. *Act of Institutional Conscience...*, p. 80-81.

In the next chapter I shall report on my empirical study of the views of physicians regarding the importance of conscience in their profession. This builds upon the previous several chapters' theoretical and historic investigation of conscience rights for health care workers. It provides some understanding of current perceptions "from the trenches" of health care provision. Unfortunately, it highlights an impression among these physicians that threats to their consciences have increased rather than decreased over the years.

CHAPTER FIVE:

EMPIRICAL STUDY OF THE PERCEPTION OF CONSCIENCE RIGHTS AMONG CHRISTIAN MEDICAL FELLOWSHIP (CMF) UK MEMBERS

The Christian Medical Fellowship (CMF) is based in the United Kingdom (UK) and currently has over 4,000 doctors and 800 medical students as members with the stated purpose of uniting and equipping Christian doctors.[421] CMF began in the UK in 1949 as a founding member of the International Christian Medical and Dental Association (ICMDA), which draws together associations from around 70 countries divided into 12 regions. CMF is actively involved in medical ethics issues and public policy work in the UK and takes policy positions in favor of conscience rights.[422] The CEO of CMF UK, Dr. Peter Saunders, is a strong advocate for conscience rights in health care and states: "Freedom of conscience is not a minor or peripheral issue. It goes to the heart of medical practice as a moral activity. Current UK law and professional guidelines respect the right of doctors to refuse to engage in certain procedures to which they have a conscientious objection. The right of conscience helps to preserve the moral integrity of the individual clinician, preserves the distinctive characteristics and reputation of medicine as a profession, acts as a safeguard against coercive state power, and provides protection from discrimination for those with minority ethical beliefs. It is worth fighting for".[423]

5.1. Aim of the Study

The aim of this empirical study was to obtain a better understanding of the perceptions of conscience rights among practicing Christian physicians. The use of questions previously employed in conscience surveys of medical doctors also allowed a basis of comparison with other studies.

---

421 CHRISTIAN MEDICAL FELLOWSHIP UK. *About. London*; (accessed on 24.11.2014, at: http://www.cmf.org.uk/about/).

422 Id. *Introducing Christian Medical Fellowship*. p. 11. London; (accessed on 24.11.2014, at: http://content.yudu.com/Library/A26zqv/IntroducingCMF/resources/index.htm?referrerUrl=http%3A%2F%2Fwww.cmf.org.uk%2Fabout%2F).

423 SAUNDERS P. *Freedom of Conscience in Medicine is Under Sustained Attack but is Worth Fighting for* (16 June 2014). London; 2014 (accessed on 22.11.2014, at: http://pjsaunders.blogspot.it/2014/06/freedom-of-conscience-in-medicine-is.html).

5.2 Methods

The study was conducted continuously from October 1, 2014 to November 17, 2014. CMF emailed an invitation to the conscience survey[424] to their entire mailing list of active physicians which consisted in 2,992 email addresses. The questionnaire was completed anonymously by respondents using a hyperlink to a virtual file which collected the responses. The survey consisted of two parts. In the first section seven closed-ended questions on the respondent's views on conscience and medical doctors. The sequence of questions two-five was randomly mixed for respondents. The second part of the questionnaire consisted of five demographic characteristics questions.[425] A "reminder email" was sent to CMF members on 4 November 2014.[426] The statistical analysis was carried out using IBM SPSS Statistical Package for the Social Sciences software.

Ethics committee approval was not required for this study.

5.3 Results

Due to invalid or wrong email addresses, 60 out 2,992 CMF members did not receive the invitation leaving 2,932 delivered to the intended recipients. A total of 843 CMF members completed all the questions and so were included in the results. The response rate was 28.75% of 2,932 delivered emails. Though a reasonable response rate is difficult to calculate without referencing a previous study using identical methodology, the 28.75% response rate for this study surpasses the 10%-20% mark typically achieved by online membership surveys.[427]

The 843 respondents were 53% female and 47% male. They fell into the age ranges; 26% 18-34, 24% 35-44, 23% 45-54, 20% 55-64, 6% 65+. Demographic question number three on ethnicity revealed overwhelming White/Caucasian background, (92%) and 2% Black, 2% Asian, 3% Other and 1% Declined to state. The question on medical specialty revealed a preponderance of Family Practice physicians, (42%) and 12% Medicine Subspecialty, 11% General Medicine, 8% Paediatrics, 6% Surgery, 6% Anaesthesiology, 4% Psychiatry, 2% Obstetrics and Gynecology, 1% Diagnostic Pathology & Radiology, 1% Non-Clinical and 7% Other. The final demographic question ascertained the years of medical practice of the respondents, and it revealed a preponderance of experienced doctors; (36%) with more than 25 years practice, 11% 21-25; 10% 16-20; 13% 11-15; 13% 6-10; 14% 1-5 and 3% less than one year's work experience.[428]

---

424 See APPENDIX A. *Survey Invitation Email*. 1 October 2014.

425 See APPENDIX B. *Online Survey of CMF UK Membership*. 1 October to 17 November 2014.

426 See APPENDIX C. *Survey Reminder Email*. 4 November 2014.

427 KNOWLEDGE BASE. *What is a Normal Survey Response Rate?*. (accessed on 22.11.2014, at: http://support2.constantcontact.com/articles/FAQ/2344).

428 APPENDIX B. *Online Survey of CMF…*, p. 3-6.

429 Due to rounding to the nearest percentage point, the addition of all the numbers may not equal 100%.

5.3.1. Analysis of Findings

On question number one, "In your opinion, how important is it to make sure that health care professionals are not forced to participate in procedures or practices to which they have moral objections?", virtually all (96%) of those surveyed stated that it is "very important" to ensure conscience protections in their professional work. The remaining 4% said this was "somewhat important" and less than 0.5% of the respondents thought it "not too important" or "not at all important

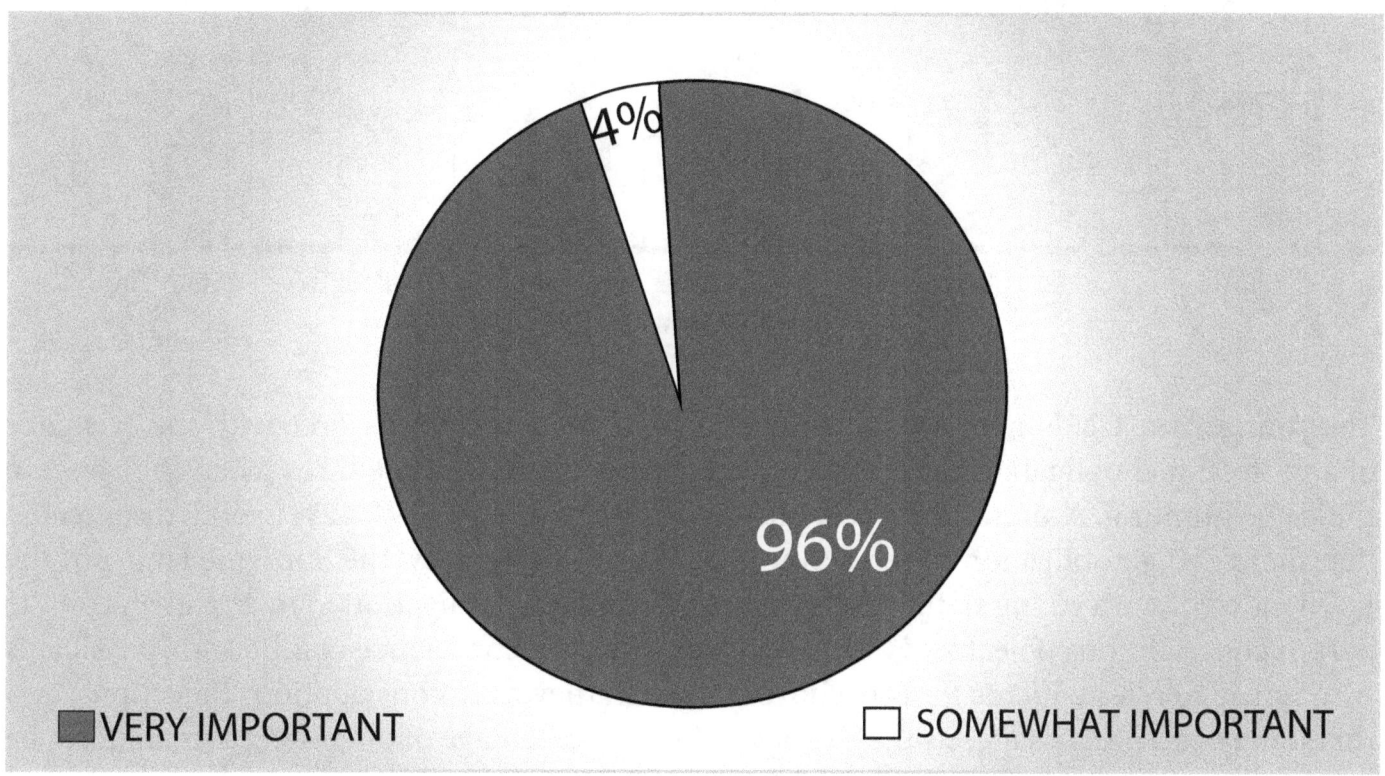

There was also near unanimity on the question, "A physician should never do what he or she believes is morally wrong, no matter what experts say" (87%). There was very little variation inresponses between less and more experienced doctors with 58% agreeing "strongly" and 29% "somewhat agreeing" while 12% disagreed, with (9%) "somewhat" and (3%) "strongly".

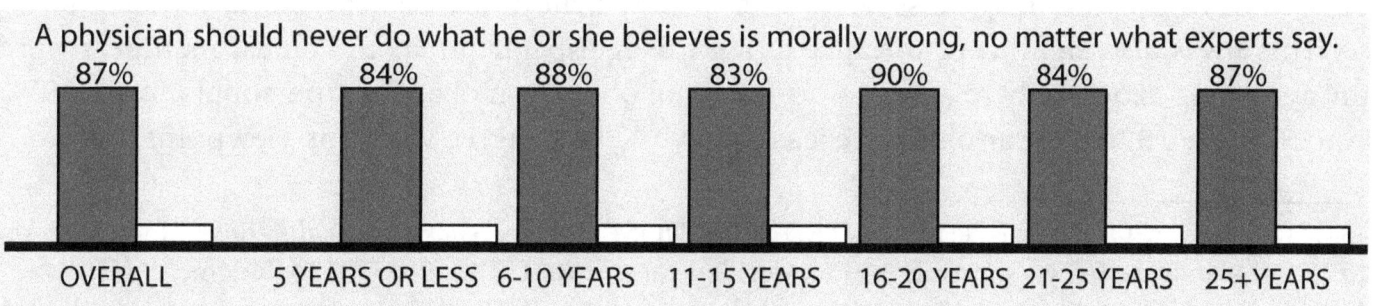

A sharp split in opinions emerged on the question, "Physicians have a professional obligation to refer patients for all legal medical services for which the patients are candidates, even if the physician believes that such a referral is immoral". Where the professional's conscience rights end and where the patient's care requirements begin was murky. 53% of CMF doctors "agreed" while 42% "disagreed" and 4% "were not sure", and these responses were broadly similar across medical specialties.

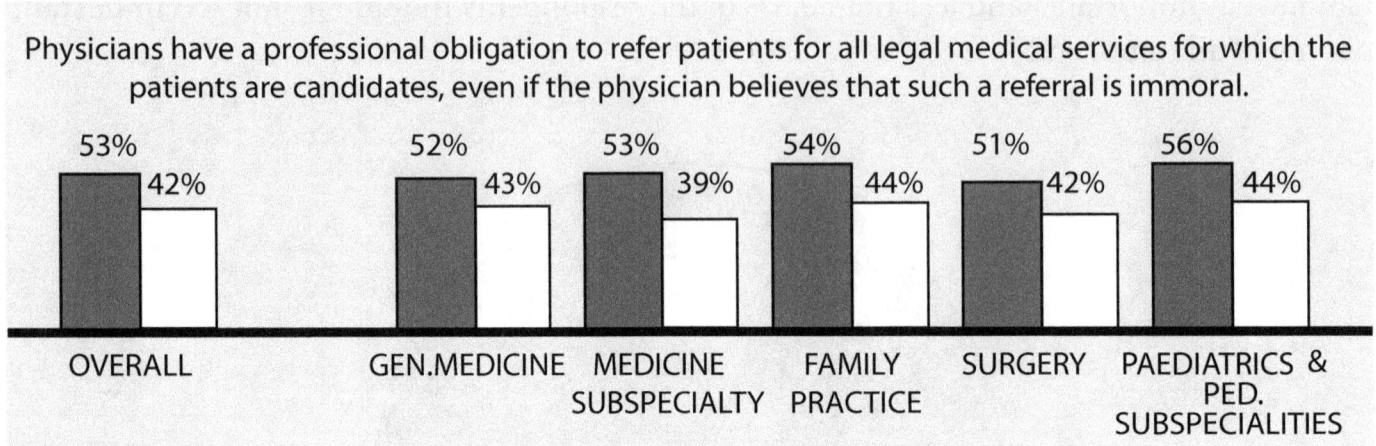

Physicians have a professional obligation to refer patients for all legal medical services for which the patients are candidates, even if the physician believes that such a referral is immoral.

The younger the CMF member, the more likely he or she was to disagree with the existence of a professional obligation to refer patients for objectionable procedures when they believe this to be immoral. Among 18-34 year olds, it was 50% "disagree" vs. 42% overall disagreeing that there was an obligation to refer. Since the time of the survey, the Supreme Court of the UK handed down a ruling stating that there is a professional obligation to refer patients on the part of conscientious objectors.[430] This decision will cause conscience conflicts for physicians who refuse to refer patients for procedures to which they have conscientious objections, and this survey and others suggests they are a significant percentage of doctors.[431] It remains to be seen if a requirement to refer will now be enforced in the United Kingdom

A second, related question also revealed a bifurcation of opinion. Members tend to disagree - albeit slightly and short of a majority – that "sometimes physicians have a professional ethical obligation to provide medical services even if they personally believe it would be morally wrong to do so" (49% disagree vs. 46% agree). CMF members with a subspecialty in medicine are more likely than average to "disagree" (57% vs. 49% overall) that physicians have an ethical obligation to provide medical services even if they believe it would be morally wrong to do so. There was also significant variance along the age spectrum, as the oldest members were the age group most likely to accept a professional obligation over their personal morals (62% agree), while 18 to 34 year olds were least likely (42%) to agree with this viewpoint.

---

430 SUPREME COURT OF THE UNITED KINGDOM. *Greater Glasgow Health Board* (accessed on 29.12.2014, at: https://www.supremecourt.uk/decided-cases/docs/UKSC_2013_0124_Judgment.pdf).
431 An American study found 43% of US physicians refuse to refer patients for procedures to which they have ethical objections. COMBS MP, ANTIEL RM, TILBURT JC, ET AL. *Conscientious Refusals to Refer...*, p. 400.

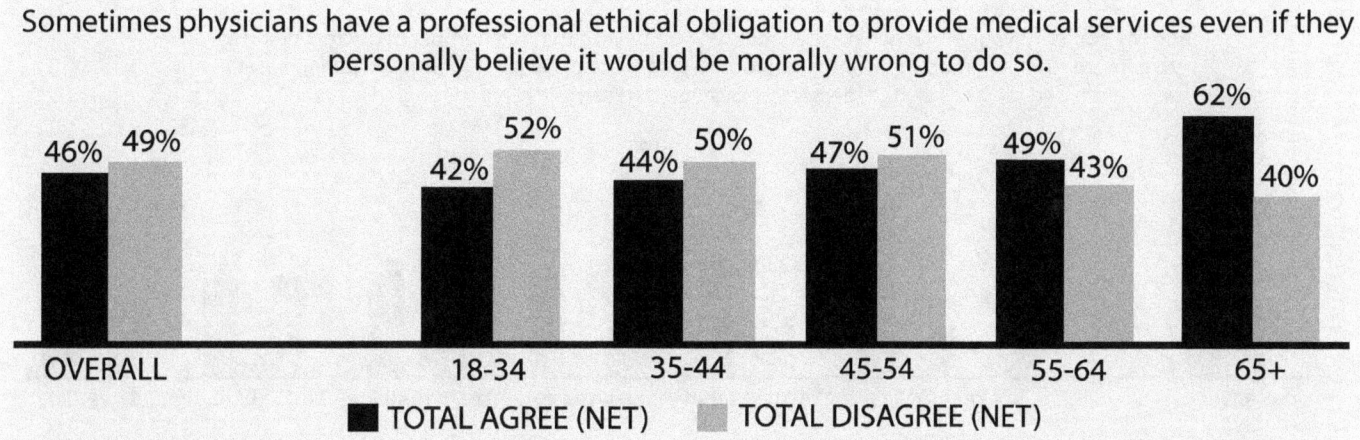

Sometimes physicians have a professional ethical obligation to provide medical services even if they personally believe it would be morally wrong to do so.

OVERALL: 46% / 49%
18-34: 42% / 52%
35-44: 44% / 50%
45-54: 47% / 51%
55-64: 49% / 43%
65+: 62% / 40%

■ TOTAL AGREE (NET) ▪ TOTAL DISAGREE (NET)

Consensus also came uneasily when CMF members were asked if they had selected their medical specialty in order to steer clear of morally abhorrent procedures. A slim majority overall (52%) disagreed. A substantial minority, 43% admitted that this was a factor in their educational calculus. The youngest set of CMF members (18 to 34 year olds) were more likely to agree (53% agree vs. 43% overall) that avoiding objectionable procedures played a role in their choice of medical specialty. Women also agreed significantly more (49%) than men (37%).

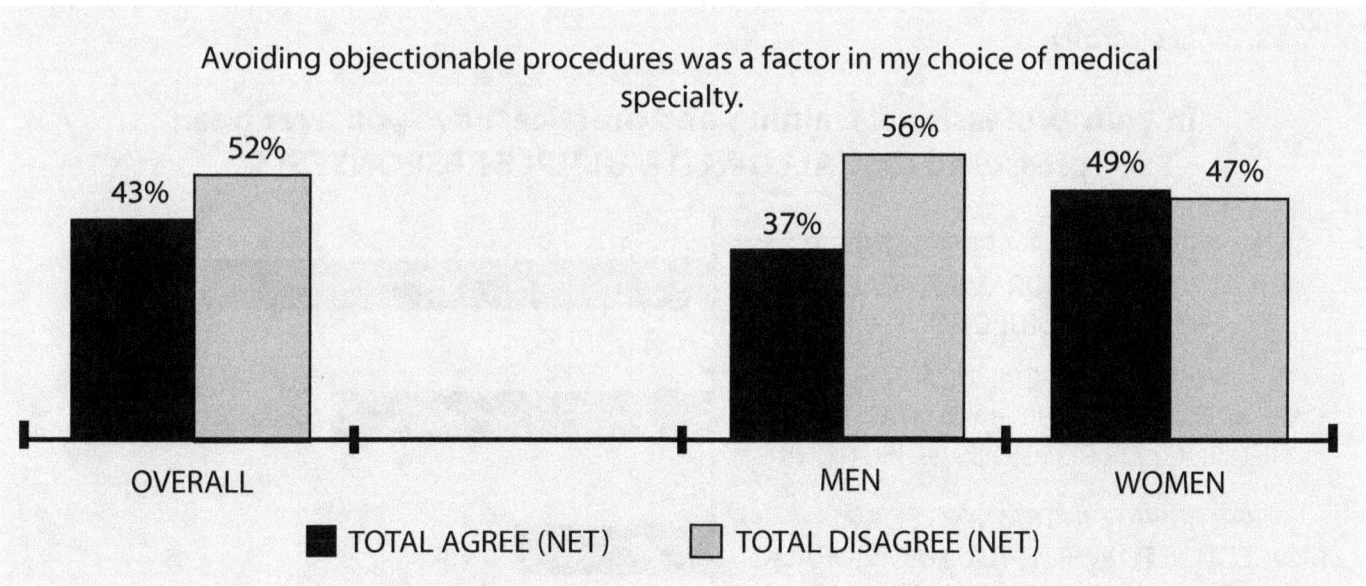

Avoiding objectionable procedures was a factor in my choice of medical specialty.

OVERALL: 43% / 52%
MEN: 37% / 56%
WOMEN: 49% / 47%

■ TOTAL AGREE (NET) □ TOTAL DISAGREE (NET)

CMF respondents believe (51%) that the number of doctors in the UK being asked to compromise their beliefs is increasing and only 2% think the number is decreasing. Members with lengthier medical careers (ages 65+) were especially likely to detect an increase in challenges to their moral, ethical or religious beliefs during the course of their careers (55% "increase" vs. 51% overall). Younger professionals were less likely to identify an increase in compromising situations, but 44% of doctors with five years or less experience selected "do not know" / "cannot judge" vs. 29% overall.

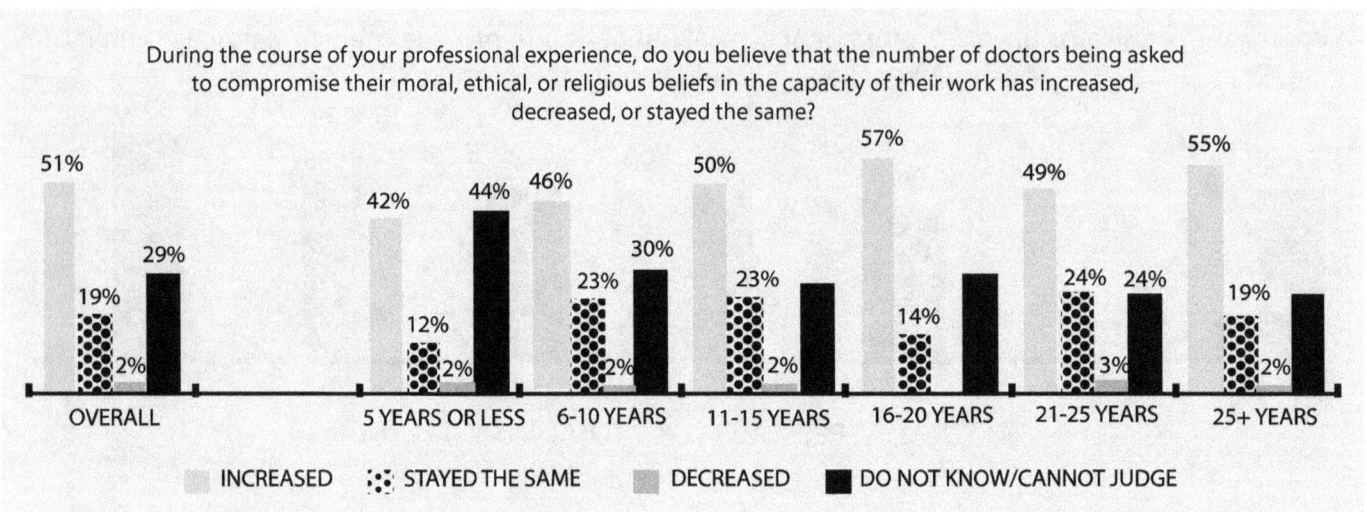

During the course of your professional experience, do you believe that the number of doctors being asked to compromise their moral, ethical, or religious beliefs in the capacity of their work has increased, decreased, or stayed the same?
51%
19%
2%
29%
42%
12%
2%
44%
46%
23%
2%
30%
50%
23%
2%
57%
14%
49%
24%
3%
24%
55%
19%
2%
OVERALL
5 YEARS OR LESS
6-10 YEARS
11-15 YEARS
16-20 YEARS
21-25 YEARS
25+ YEARS
INCREASED
STAYED THE SAME
DECREASED
DO NOT KNOW/CANNOT JUDGE

On the final question, multiple answers were permitted. Over half of CMF members (54%) were recipients of pressure that went against their moral, ethical or religious values. This burden is felt most acutely in the area of being asked to "refer a patient for a procedure to which [they] had moral, ethical, or religious objections" (37%). Pressure to prescribe for a patient a medication to which they object was the next highest issue (28%). Members specializing in "family practice", the largest category (42%), were considerably more likely to be pressured to refer patients for a procedure toward which they held personal objections (60% vs. 37% overall).

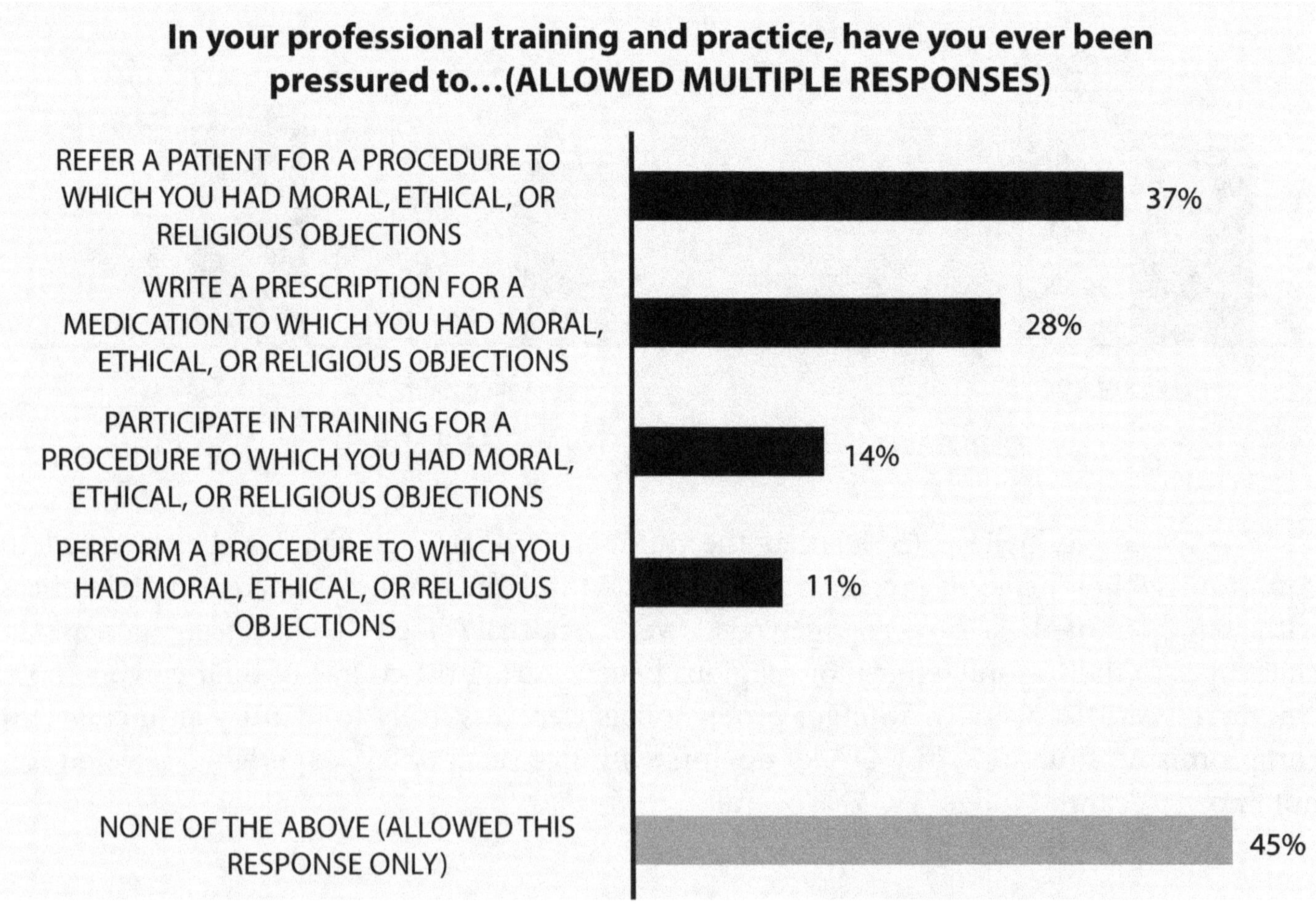

In your professional training and practice, have you ever been pressured to...(ALLOWED MULTIPLE RESPONSES)
REFER A PATIENT FOR A PROCEDURE TO WHICH YOU HAD MORAL, ETHICAL, OR RELIGIOUS OBJECTIONS
37%
WRITE A PRESCRIPTION FOR A MEDICATION TO WHICH YOU HAD MORAL, ETHICAL, OR RELIGIOUS OBJECTIONS
28%
PARTICIPATE IN TRAINING FOR A PROCEDURE TO WHICH YOU HAD MORAL, ETHICAL, OR RELIGIOUS OBJECTIONS
14%
PERFORM A PROCEDURE TO WHICH YOU HAD MORAL, ETHICAL, OR RELIGIOUS OBJECTIONS
11%
NONE OF THE ABOVE (ALLOWED THIS RESPONSE ONLY)
45%

5.4 Discussion

CMF UK members share a nearly unanimous belief in the great importance of conscience protections for medical professionals. The results of the study revealed a considerable division of opinion, however, when moving into the concrete conscience problems of health care delivery. Overall 53% agreed to there being a professional obligation to refer, even if the physician believes that such a referral is immoral. This does not square easily with the 87% who responded that physicians should never do what is morally wrong, no matter what experts say. It is possible that there was some confusion concerning the morality of referral in general for a procedure to which a health care worker objects.[432] The findings were consistent with Combs, Antiel, Tilburt, ET AL's 57% agree from 2,000 randomly selected US physicians from all specialties who were asked the same question.[433] It also correlates with their observation that more religious and more conservative physicians are less likely to be willing to refer patients for objectionable procedures.[434] The similarities in the results are all the more interesting given the different societal and medical cultures in the UK and the USA.

The limitations of this study nevertheless include the fact that it focused only on practicing Christian doctors in the UK belonging to one major organization and was reliant on self-selection such that there could be response bias. The 53% of females among the respondents is higher than the 47% of women among British doctors in 2012, but the trend is toward ever greater percentages of women physicians.[435] The study utilized the entire email list of CMF active physician members with accessible emails, but this proved to be only 2,932 out of over 4,000+ CMF members, and the response rate of 28.75% translates into an estimated margin of error of ±3.1%.

The Christian Medical & Dental Associations (CMDA), the US affiliate of the ICMDA to which CMF UK belongs, did an electronic survey on conscience rights among their members, the Catholic Medical Association, the Fellowship of Christian Physicians Assistants, Christian

---

432 The internal CMF division on the broader referral issue is reflected in articles and letters highlighting the different approaches of several CMF doctors and not taking a clear-cut institutional position in their journal. FERGUSSON A. *Abortion Requests: Should We 'Refer'?*. Triple Helix. 2010; Easter: 14-15 (accessed on 23.11.2014, at: http://admin.cmf.org.uk/pdf/helix/spr10/th-spr10p14-15.pdf); DAVIES P. *Abortion Referrals*. Triple Helix. 2010; Summer: 21 (accessed on 23.11.2014, at: http://admin.cmf.org. uk/pdf/helix/sum10/THsum10p20-21.pdf).

433 COMBS MP, ANTIEL RM, TILBURT JC, ET AL. *Conscientious Refusals to Refer: Findings from a National Physician Survey*. J Med Ethics. 2011; 37: 397-401, p. 397.

434 *Ibid.* p. 399

435 MEIRON THOMAS J. *Why Having so Many Women Doctors is Hurting the NHS: A Provocative but Powerful Argument from a Leading Surgeon*. Mail Online (2 January 2014). London; 2014 (accessed on 24.11.2014, at: http://www.dailymail.co.uk/debate/article-2532461/Why-having-women-doctors-hurting-NHS-A-provovcative-powerful-argument-leading-surgeon.html).

Pharmacists Fellowship International and Nurses Christian Fellowship in 2009.[436] They received an almost identical overwhelming response on the importance of conscience protections, (97% agree vs. almost 100% CMF). CMDA asked questions regarding professional pressures which I used in my CMF survey with lower but similar responses concerning pressure to refer, (32% vs. 37%) and pressure to prescribe, (26% vs. 28%).[437] The US responders, however, felt slightly more pressure to undergo training for an objectionable procedure, (17% vs. 14%) and to perform a procedure to which they object (12% vs. 11%).[438] Once again, the similarity of results obtained from the same questions in the UK and the USA is striking.

There were, however, significant differences in results from the CMF study and Lawrence and Curlin's US survey mailed in 2007 with two of the same questions. The US study recorded 78% physicians responding that they are never obligated to do what they believe to be wrong vs. 87% in the CMF study.[439] Then 57% agreed that they sometimes have an ethical obligation to provide services they believe to be morally wrong vs. 46% among CMF members.[440] Lawrence and Curlin were also surprised by the overlap in answers to what should have been mutually incompatible statements, and they might have reacted to the different ways they were formulated or that they share prima facie commitments to both conscience and professional obligations.[441] I believe that a significant number of doctors have a hard time believing their profession could require something unethical of them and so they intellectually submit to obligations that they otherwise would see as morally wrong. I agree with Lawrence and Curlin that further research to clarify these ambiguities is warranted.

5.5 Conclusions

This CMF UK perception of conscience rights study gives a snapshot of a troubling situation in the modern health sector. CMF members are highly aware of and concerned about the coercion of doctor's consciences. They experience the problem as growing in intensity.

The tremendous difference between those who see pressure on doctors to compromise beliefs at work as increasing, (51%) as opposed to decreasing (2%) is perhaps the most striking finding of the CMF study. These results become even more dramatic when adjusted for experience in health care work. The oldest physicians were much more likely to see the

---

436 IMBODY J. *Data and Analysis of Two National Surveys on Conscience Rights Regulation and Laws, as Related to HHS Requested Information on Rescission Proposal.* CMDA (9 April 2009). Bristol: 2009: p. 4. (accessed on 24.11.2014, at: http://cmda.org/library/doclib/cma-survey-analysis-for-hhs.pdf).
437 *Ibid.* p. 8.
438 *Ibid.*
439 The 56% for Evangelicals was nevertheless much higher than the agreement from doctors with noreligion, (33%). LAWRENCE RE, CURLIN FA. *Physicians' Beliefs About Conscience in Medicine: A National Survey.* Acad Med. 2009; 84 (9): 1276-1282, p. 1279.
440 *Ibid.*
441 *Ibid.* p. 1281.

situation as deteriorating, (55%) than were the youngest, (42%). This points to a real and deepening crisis of conscience in the health care sector, especially when combined with the substantial minority of doctors who took into account objectionable procedures in choosing a medical specialty, (43%).

At the same time, about half see themselves as obligated to refer patients against their will and even to provide objectionable medical services. These kinds of pressures are a part of the professional lives of a majority, (54%), of those surveyed, and a substantial minority chose their medical specialties keeping potential conscience difficulties in mind.

It is not unrealistic to see medicine as becoming more and more inhospitable, or even inaccessible in certain specialties, to "Hippocratic doctors" in the near future in certain countries if positive changes are not made.[442]

---

442 My heartfelt thanks go to Dr. Peter Saunders and Martin Parsons from CMF UK for giving permission for and facilitating this study. I also wish to thank Kevin Quinley and Kellyanne Conway from the polling company, inc./Woman Trend.

CONCLUSION

Conscience, even when limited to the sphere of health care workers, is a vast topic. My objective in this dissertation has been to analyze why it is so essentially important to respect and foster the moral integrity of all those involved in the healing professions. It is a true and felicitous phrase that medicine is a moral enterprise[443] intimately involved in many of the most dramatic moments of human life. Society looks to medicine as it does to law and religion to validate what is ethical and desirable. The modern problem of conscience conflicts and health workers involves many elements, and I tried to examine the most relevant ones for a bioethical analysis.

During the twentieth century, a major change took place in medical ethics. The traditional model of health care delivery, now termed medical paternalism, involved the doctor or health professional making all major treatment decisions with the patient simply expected to cooperate with the course of action deemed best by the professionals. This model was heavily dependent on faith in the beneficence of health workers and the higher quality of their decisions for the benefit of the patient. This faith was deeply shaken by the shocking revelations of science and medicine as ruthless instruments of a totalitarian state during World War II and other scandals such as the Tuskegee Syphilis Study by the U.S. Public Health Service.[444]

A new model emphasizing the informed consent and the autonomy of patients became increasingly dominant. A seminal moment in this process was the Belmont Report in 1979 and the new regulations and legislation governing experimentation involving human subjects that were put into place. The patient's rights to informed consent are now so entrenched that it is even controversial to perform emergency research that might prove beneficial to the patient because obtaining consent is frequently impossible in emergency situations. The opposite side of this coin is that doctors and other medical professionals, who used to be unquestioned decision-makers, can now be almost reduced to "a role of morally neutral technicians" which violates the whole idea of medical ethics.[445] "Forcing a physician to violate his conscience breaks this bond of trust and indicates an inequality of freedom within the relationship, thus destroying the foundation for the principle of autonomy".[446]

---

443 PELLEGRINO. *The Medical Profession...*, p. 222.

444 REVERBY SM. *More Than Fact and Fiction: Cultural Memory and the Tuskegee Syphilis Study*. Hastings Cent Rep. 2001; 31 (5): 22-28, p. 22.

445 PELLEGRINO ED. *Societal Duty and Moral Complicity: The Physician's Dilemma of Divided Loyalty*. Int J Law Psychiatry. 1993; 16: 371-391, p. 381.

446 BURKE. *The Loss of a Physician's...*, p. 418.

On top of this sea change in the doctor-patient relationship there was a major change in morality in the West in the latter half of the twentieth century, often called the Sexual Revolution. In the space of only a few decades, contraception and sterilization went from being commonly legally prohibited to a widespread practice sanctioned by court rulings and laws in dozens of countries. Abortion followed a similar trajectory. The rapid pace of social and legal change continues to this day with the legalization of euthanasia and physician assisted suicide in several countries and increasing social pressure to do so in many others. Doctors who started medical school in the 1950s found themselves confronted later in their careers with patients demanding a whole range of procedures that did not exist or were not only considered unethical but were legally banned when they began to practice. It is no wonder that so many health professionals feel ethically assaulted and refuse in conscience to collaborate in many of these procedures.

My empirical study for this dissertation of physician members of the Christian Medical Fellowship in the UK confirmed what several other studies have found, that there is a perceived problem of growing threats to conscience for health care providers today.[447] While 96% of respondents agreed it was "very important" to ensure they have conscience protections in their professional work so that they are not forced to participate in procedures or practices to which they have moral objections, 51% said the number of doctors being asked to compromise their moral, ethical, or religious beliefs in the capacity of their work has increased.[448] Only 2% thought the numbers had decreased. Even more troubling, 43% agreed that avoiding objectionable procedures was a factor in their choice of medical specialty.[449] Clearly, the process of selecting out individuals with conscientious objections to certain procedures from certain medical specialties is well advanced.

Technological and scientific discoveries have also created new conscience quandaries, particularly with regards to newly possible manipulations of the recently conceived human embryo. In vitro fertilization and the killing of human embryos by the extraction of their stem cells for scientific research have opened a Pandora's Box of ethical problems that increasingly affect scientists and health workers in many specialties. New drugs with potentially abortifacient characteristics have become commonly available, and at the same time legal pressure on pharmacists and other health professionals to providethese drugs has increased.

---

447 See Chapter 5 for in-depth discussion of this study.

448 57% of physicians with 16-20 years experience responded that more doctors are being asked to compromise their consciences while only 42% doctors with 5 or less years experience said the same, suggesting that pressure on conscience has increased over time.

449 12% of those strongly agreed and 31% somewhat agreed.

Contemporary medicine is many times more powerful than it was even a few decades ago. Technological advances applied to the life sciences are happening at a blindingly fast rate. Never has it been truer that ethical restraint and moral wisdom are required. As the proverbial wisdom puts it, "just because we can do something doesn't mean that we should do it". Resisting the tremendous temptation for scientists and health care professionals to "play God" is an important aspect of conscience in medicine. "When physicians peaceably refuse to participate in some new moral project involving the application of medical science, they stand witnesses to the intrinsic connections between science and ethics in the practice of medicine. They help to bring our norms out into the open, and they force us to ask and to debate many important questions".[450] We need more conscience not less in medicine today even if it makes the process of health care delivery more complicated. Medical students, in particular, are in urgent need of assistance in properly forming their consciences in line with objective criteria.

The worst case ethical scenario is the combination of a Totalitarian State wielding science and medicine as weapons in a will to power that crushes all opposition.[451] Historically, medical professionals and others with strong consciences were the only effective means of internal resistance to an all-powerful State which controlled all institutions and enforced its will on society. There are also much less extreme scenarios that are nevertheless of urgent concern today. Activist organizations, mainly Radical Feminist and "Sexual and Reproductive Health" oriented groups, have targeted conscience protections for health care workers and institutions for reduction/elimination around the world. Their overwhelming concern is increased access to abortion, and even the most reasonable accommodations of the conscience rights of health care providers are suspect to them. They are alarmed that more rather than less health professionals have taken the route of conscientious objection to abortion and other procedures in recent years. Lawsuits and proposed legislative and regulatory changes have been part of their attacks on conscience rights.

Another particularly worrying aspect of the modern health care scene concerns certain anti-conscience campaigns that primarily target the Catholic Church's health care institutions. A prime example is the "Merger Watch" initiative.[452] It is clear that these groups would prefer that Catholic hospitals close or not be allowed to merge with other institutions, with all the negative health consequences this could entail on local communities, rather than allowing them to refrain from permitting a very limited range of controversial procedures. It is reasonable to posit that an anti-religious animus, specifically anti-Catholicism, is motivating at least some of these attacks. The enormous controversy and myriad court cases concerning the Obama Administration's attempt to force many employers and individuals to pay for

---

450 ELSHTAIN JB. *Why Science Cannot Stand Alone.* Theor Med Bioeth. 2008; 29: 161-169, p. 167.
451 *Ibid.* p. 168.
452 MERGER WATCH. *In Medical Care…*, (accessed on 22.11.2014, at: http://www.mergerwatch.org/about/).

contraceptives and potentially abortifacient birth control in health insurance coverage, despite strong religious and conscientious objections, is a clear sign that a societal crisis of conscience in the health care sector is unfolding in the USA.

Therefore, it is urgently necessary for academics in the field of bioethics to analyze the importance of the role of conscience in health care provision. In this dissertation, I attempted to show why it is not a groundless demand for special treatment to require respect for manifestations of conscience by health workers such as certain cases of medical conscientious objection. It is acceptable to investigate if objections proceed from a command of conscience or from another source, but we should not lose site of the fact that individuals truly have a non-negotiable duty to follow the judgments of their consciences.[453] "The physician as a human being has the same claim to respect for his or her capacity to make moral choices, to follow his or her conscience about what is good medicine and what is morally acceptable as a person".[454] The personal integrity of health workers should be protected when their conscientious beliefs are reasonable, especially in view of the fact that doctors are not required to provide all possible interventions and something as simple as lack of interest can justify not offering a procedure.[455]

Certainly, a prerequisite is to have a proper grasp of the nature of conscience, which I wrote about in the first chapter. It is also important to understand the ends of medicine, which were once clear to virtually all thanks to the Hippocratic Tradition. Unfortunately, principles like "first do no harm" and the prohibitions on doctors taking human lives are increasingly challenged or rejected today. This makes the bulwark of conscience protections all the more important if it is ethically unacceptable for the medical professions to be systematically purged of adherents to the Hippocratic Tradition. It is particularly ironic that in an age which extols "diversity" and "tolerance", divergent views that would benefit from conscience protections are attacked in favor of the imposition of a single "orthodox" liberal ethical view of controversial procedures and even what constitute the ends of medicine. The new "enemies of conscience" falsely claim that conscientious objectors "coerce" patients or "impose" their beliefs on them, but actually the reverse happens more frequently, namely coercing doctors to violate their consciences.[456]

---

453 KANTYMIR L, MCLEOD C. *Justification for Conscience Exemptions in Health Care.* Bioethics. 2014; 28 (1): 16-23, p. 16-17.

454 PELLEGRINO ED. *Patient and Physician Autonomy: Conflicting Rights and Obligations in the Physician-Patient Relationship.* J Contemp Health Law Policy.1994; 10: 47-68, p. 51.

455 KACZOR K. *Abortion, Conscience, and Doctors* (29 October 2010). Princeton; 2010 (accessed on 24.11.2014, at: http://www.thepublicdiscourse.com/2010/10/1922/).

456 GEORGE. *Conscience and its Enemies*, p. 159.

Moral integrity is a fundamental good and its opposite a terrible evil. Policies, regulations or laws that force medical professionals to violate their consciences lead inevitably to one consequence, the elimination of whole categories of moral individuals from the medical field. They will either be forced to resign from their profession or become morally compromised by collaborating in what they believe to be evil. This potential state of affairs is a stark prospect. Scholars rightfully point out the risks as negatively influencing the type of persons choosing to study medicine, "moral divestiture", "callousness", diminished sympathy for patient's diverse moral beliefs and lack of loyalty and fidelity to professional responsibilities.[457]

In conclusion, I assert that conscience is a fundamental right for all individuals and should be respected. The health professions are especially vulnerable to attempts at undermining conscience as a consequence of certain aggressive ideological positions, particularly those advocating the admissibility of taking innocent human lives. If the frequently re-affirmed fundamental human right to conscience and the modern human rights regime are to remain meaningful, the rolling back of conscience protections for health care workers and institutions must be rejected. We should also remember the negative lessons of recent history when conscience was trampled upon by Totalitarian States, and see the practical safeguards inherent in respecting conscience in all areas of society, but particularly in health care. That is not to affirm that reasonable limitations may not be placed on some expressions of conscience since it is generally acknowledged that this faculty is fallible. Nevertheless, denying conscience rights is the antithesis of ethical acting, and only particularly weighty reasons can justify curbs on these rights. This is particularly true in the moral enterprise that is medicine.

---

457 WHITE, BRODY. *Would Accommodating...*, p. 1804-1805

APPENDIX A:
SURVEY INVITATION EMAIL

October 1, 2014

RE: Invitation to the CMF Membership Study

Dear CMF Member,

The Christian Medical Fellowship and a doctoral candidate are conducting a short survey among CMF UK members on their experiences and opinions regarding conscience rights in health care. They have commissioned the polling company, inc., a market research firm based in Washington, D.C., to administer this study.

The survey will be available to take online for a brief period. The survey will take approximately 5 minutes to complete and can be taken at any time of day using any computer with internet access.

All responses will be kept confidential, and all identifying information will be removed from the data, and results will only be shared in aggregate.

Please complete the survey by clicking the link below and following the instructions from there:

{SurveyLink}

If the above link is not "live," please copy and paste the full address into a web browser. When copying and pasting the link, if necessary, please ensure that there are no spaces or punctuation following the address, and that you have copied the entire link, including the letter or number characters at the end.

If you have any problems accessing or completing the online survey, please contact the polling company, inc. at survey@pollingcompany.com.

Thank you in advance for your help.

Christian Medical Fellowship
the polling company, inc.

APPENDIX B:
ONLINE SURVEY OF CMF UK MEMBERSHIP

Field Dates: October 1 – November 17, 2014
Margin of Error: ±3.1% 843 participants 28.75% response rate

1. In your opinion, how important is it to make sure that healthcare professionals are not forced to participate in procedures or practices to which they have moral objections?

   96% VERY IMPORTANT
   4% SOMEWHAT IMPORTANT
   * NOT TOO IMPORTANT
   * NOT AT ALL IMPORTANT
   1% DO NOT KNOW/IT DEPENDS

Next, you will read a series of statements about conscience protections for physicians. For each, please select whether you (ROTATED) agree or disagree with that statement. (RANDOMIZED SEQUENCE)

2. Physicians have a professional obligation to refer patients for all legal medical services for which the patients are candidates, even if the physician believes that such a referral is immoral.

   53% TOTAL AGREE (NET)
   18% STRONGLY AGREE
   35% SOMEWHAT AGREE

   42% TOTAL DISAGREE (NET)
   20% SOMEWHAT DISAGREE
   23% STRONGLY DISAGREE

   4% DO NOT KNOW/NOT SURE

3. A physician should never do what he or she believes is morally wrong, no matter what experts say.

   87% TOTAL AGREE (NET)
   58% STRONGLY AGREE
   29% SOMEWHAT AGREE

   12% TOTAL DISAGREE (NET)
   9% SOMEWHAT DISAGREE
   3% STRONGLY DISAGREE

1% DO NOT KNOW/NOT SURE

4. Sometimes physicians have a professional ethical obligation to provide medical services even if they personally believe it would be morally wrong to do so.

46% TOTAL AGREE (NET)
8% STRONGLY AGREE
38% SOMEWHAT AGREE

49% TOTAL DISAGREE (NET)
20% SOMEWHAT DISAGREE
29% STRONGLY DISAGREE

5% DO NOT KNOW/NOT SURE

5. Avoiding objectionable procedures was a factor in my choice of medical specialty.

43% TOTAL AGREE (NET)
12% STRONGLY AGREE
31% SOMEWHAT AGREE

52% TOTAL DISAGREE (NET)
20% SOMEWHAT DISAGREE
32% STRONGLY DISAGREE

5% DO NOT KNOW/NOT SURE

(ENDED RANDOMIZE)

6. During the course of your professional experience, do you believe that the number of doctors being asked to compromise their moral, ethical, or religious beliefs in thecapacity of their work has increased, decreased, or stayed the same?

51% INCREASED
19% STAYED THE SAME
2% DECREASED
29% DO NOT KNOW/CANNOT JUDGE

7. In your professional training and practice, have you ever been pressured to...(ALLOWED MULTIPLE RESPONSES)

37% REFER A PATIENT FOR A PROCEDURE TO WHICH YOU HAD MORAL, ETHICAL, OR RELIGIOUS OBJECTIONS
28% WRITE A PRESCRIPTION FOR A MEDICATION TO WHICH YOU HAD MORAL, ETHICAL, OR RELIGIOUS OBJECTIONS
14% PARTICIPATE IN TRAINING FOR A PROCEDURE TO WHICH YOU HAD MORAL, ETHICAL, OR RELIGIOUS OBJECTIONS

11% PERFORM A PROCEDURE TO WHICH YOU HAD MORAL, ETHICAL, OR RELIGIOUS OBJECTIONS

45% NONE OF THE ABOVE (ALLOWED THIS RESPONSE ONLY)
1% DO NOT KNOW/CANNOT REMEMBER (ALLOWED THIS RESPONSE ONLY)

Demographics

Finally, a few questions for statistical purposes only….

8. Are you…

> 47% MALE
> 53% FEMALE

9. Into which of the following categories does your age fall?

> 26% 18-34
> 24% 35-44
> 23% 45-54
> 20% 55-64
> 6% 65+
>
> * DECLINED TO STATE

10. Which of the following best describes your ethnicity? (SINGLE RESPONSE)

> 92% WHITE/CAUCASIAN
> 2% BLACK
> 2% ASIAN
> * MIDDLE EASTERN
>
> **3% OTHER, SPECIFIED (RECORDED) (NET)**
> British and Asian
> Chinese
> Chinese
> Chinese Malaysian
> East Asian
> English/Thai
> Mixed
> Mixed white and Asian
> Oriental
> Sri Lankan
> White African
>
> * DECLINED TO STATE

11. In what specialty do you work?

42% FAMILY PRACTICE
12% MEDICINE SUBSPECIALTY
11% GENERAL MEDICINE
8% PAEDIATRICS AND PED. SUBSPECIALTIES
6% SURGERY
6% ANAESTHESIOLOGY
4% PSYCHIATRY
2% OBSTETRICS AND GYNAECOLOGY
1% DIAGNOSTIC-PATHOLOGY & RADIOLOGY
1% NON-CLINICAL

7% OTHER, SPECIFIED (RECORDED) (NET)

A&E
Clinical Oncology
Currently between jobs, just completed foundation programme
CurrentlyMedical Oncology & Palliative Medicine + worked in Surgery, Obstetrics and Gynaecology
Emergency medicine
EmergencyMedicine
EMERGENCY MEDICINE
Emergency medicine - currently on foundation rotations
F1
Family practice and psychiatry
Foundation training
Foundation training
Geriatric Medicine
Geriatrics
GP trainee currently in paediatrics but will rotate specialties 4 monthly
GP training various currently a@e
Missionary surgeon, now retired
Not a specialist yet...recently graduated
Now in public health, previously medicine for elderly
Occupational health
OccupationalMedicine
ONCOLOGY
Ophthalmology
Ophthalmology
Palliative care
Palliative medicine
Palliative medicine

Palliative Medicine
PharmaceuticalMedicine
Public health
Public Health
RespiratoryMedicine
Retired GP
Rural medicine in developing country-do all the above!
Sexual and reproductive health
Sexual and reproductive health
Sexual and Reproductive health

12. Excluding your education, for how long have you been in the medical profession?

3% LESS THAN ONE YEAR
14% 1-5 YEARS
13% 6-10 YEARS
13% 11-15 YEARS
10% 16-20 YEARS
11% 21-25 YEARS
36% MORE THAN 25 YEARS

* REFUSE TO ANSWER

APPENDIX C:
SURVEY REMINDER EMAIL

November 4, 2014

RE: Reminder to Participate in the Christian Medical Fellowship (CMF)Membership Study

Dear CMF Member:

The Christian Medical Fellowship and a doctoral candidate are conducting a short survey among CMF UK members on their experiences and opinions regarding conscience rights in health care.

On Monday, October 13, you received an email invitation to take this survey. If you have already completed the survey and submitted your response, we thank you for participating. Kindly ignore this reminder. <u>If you have not yet completed the survey, we ask that you do so by Friday, November 14.</u>

The survey will take approximately 5 minutes to complete and can be taken conveniently at any time of day using any computer with Internet access.

All responses will be kept confidential, and all identifying information will be removed from the data, and results will only be shared in aggregate. To ensure these protocols, CMF has contracted with a US-based research firm in its 20th year of operation.

Please complete the survey by clicking the link below and following the instructions from there:

{SurveyLink}

If the above link is not "live," please copy and paste the full address into a web browser. When copying and pasting the link, if necessary, please ensure that there are no spaces or punctuation following the address, and that you have copied the entire link, including the letter or number characters at the end.

If you have any problems accessing or completing the online survey, please contact the survey administrators at survey@pollingcompany.com.

Thank you in advance for your help.

Christian Medical Fellowship &
the polling company, inc.

BIBLIOGRAPHY

ADAMS MP. *Conscience and Conflict*. Am J Bioeth. 2007; 7 (12): 28-29.

D'AGOSTINO F. *L'Obiezione di Coscienza Come Diritto*. Iustitia. 2009; 62: 177-182.

ALEXANDER L. *Medical Science Under Dictatorship*. N Engl J Med. 1949; 241 (2): 39-47.

ALTA CHARO R. *The Celestial Fire of Conscience — Refusing to Deliver Medical Care*. N Eng J Med. 2005; 352: 2471-2473.

AMERICAN ASSOCIATION OF PRO LIFE OBSTETRICIANS AND GYNECOLOGISTS (AAPLOG). *The Recent History of Conscience Rules* (26 July 2012). Eau Claire; 2012 (accessed on 24.10.2014, at: http://www.aaplog.org/physicianconscience- rights/the-recent-history-of-conscience-rules/).

AMERICAN COLLEGE OF OBSTETRICIANS AND GYNECOLOGISTS (ACOG) COMMITTEE ON ETHICS. *The Limits of Conscientious Refusal in Reproductive Medicine ACOG Committee Opinion no. 385*. Obstet Gynecol. 2007; 110: 1203-1208.

AMERICAN MEDICAL ASSOCIATION (AMA). H-120.947 *Preserving Patients'Ability to Have Legally Valid Prescriptions Filled* (18 June 2005) Chicago: 2005 (accessed on 07.08.2014, at: http://www.ama-assn.org/ad-com/polfind/ Hlth-Ethics.pdf).

AMERICAN NURSES ASSOCIATION. *Code of Ethics for Nurses With Interpretive Statements*. (15 November 2010). Silver Spring; 2010 (accessed on 22.11.2014, at: http://www.nursing world.org/MainMenuCategories/EthicsStandards/ CodeofEthicsforNurses/Code-of-Ethics. pdf).

AMERICAN NURSES ASSOCIATION. *The Nonnegotiable Nature of the ANA Code for Nurses with Interpretive Statements* (8 December 1994). Silver Spring; 1994 (accessed on 22.11.2014, at: http://nursingworld.org/MainMenuCategories/Policy-Advocacy/Positions-and-Resolutions/ ANA PositionStatements/Position-Statements-Alphabetically/ prtetcode14446.html).

AMERICAN NURSES ASSOCIATION. *What is Nursing?* (accessed on 17.10.2014, at: http:// www.nursingworld.org/EspeciallyForYou/What-is-Nursing).

AMERICAN PHARMACISTS ASSOCIATION (APhA). *Code of Ethics* (27 October 1994). Washington, D.C.; 1994 (accessed 06.08.2014, at: http://www.pharmacist.com/code-ethics).

ANDERSON N. *Pharmacists with No Plan B: Freedom of Conscience and 'Reproductive Rights' Clash at the Local Drugstore*. Christianity Today, 1 August 2006; (accessed 20.08.2014, at: http://www.christianitytoday.com/ct/2006/august/31.44.html?paging=off).

ANDREW EG. *Conscience and its Critics: Protestant Conscience, Enlightenment Reason, and Modern Subjectivity*. Toronto: University of Toronto Press; 2001.

AQUINAS T. *Summa Theologica*. English Trans. FATHERS OF THE ENGLISH DOMINICAN PROVINCE. Raleigh: Hayes Barton Press; 2006.

ARENDT H. *Eichmann in Jerusalem: A Report on the Banality of Evil*. New York: Penguin Books; 2006.

ARENDT H. *Thinking and Moral Considerations: A Lecture*. Social Research. 1971; 38 (3): 417-446.ARISTOTLE. Rhetoric. English Trans. RHYS ROBERTS W. New York: Cosimo Inc.; 2010.

ASHLEY B. *Elements of a Catholic Conscience* in SMITH RE (editor). Catholic Conscience: Foundation and Formation: Proceedings of the Tenth Bishops' Workshop, Dallas, Texas. Braintree: The Pope John XXIII Medical-Moral Research and Education Center; 1991: 39-57.

ASSOCIATION OF WOMEN'S HEALTH, OBSTETRIC & NEONATAL NURSING (AWHONN). *Ethical Decision Making in the Clinical Setting: Nurses' Rights and Responsibilities* (June 2009). Washington DC; 2009 (accessed on 22.11.2014, at: http://childrightsnurses.org/wp-content/uploads/2013/03/Resources_Documents_pdf_ 5_ Ethics-copy1.pdf).

AUGUSTINE. *Confessions of Saint Augustine*. English Trans. SHEED FJ. London: Sheed & Ward; 1984.

AUSTRIAN PARLIAMENT. *Federal Law No. 60 of 23 January 1974*. Vienna: Federal Law Gazette; 1974: (accessed on 18.07.2011, at: http://www.hsph.harvard.edu/ population/abortion/Austria.abo.htm).

BAHM AJ. *Theories of Conscience*. Ethics. 1965; 75 (2): 128-131.

BBC NEWS. *Catholic midwives win appeal over abortion case*. BBC News (24 April 2013). London; 2013 (accessed on 08.10.2014, at: http://www.bbc.com/news/ukscotland-glasgow-west-22279857).

BEAUCHAMP T, CHILDRESS J. *Principles of Biomedical Ethics*. New York: Oxford University Press; 20015.

BEDFORD EL. *The Act of Institutional Conscience: An Examination and Defense* [dissertation]. St. Louis: Saint Louis Univ.; 2014.

BEDFORD EL. *The Concept of Institutional Conscience*. Natl Cathol Bioeth Q. 2012; 12 (3): 409-429.

BELLUCK P. *Abortion Qualms on Morning-After Pill May Be Unfounded*. New York Times (5 June 2012). New York; 2012 (accessed on 25.11.2014, at; http://www.nytimes.com/2012/06/06/health/research/morning-after-pills-dont-blockimplantation-science-suggests.html?pagewanted=al l&_r=0).

BENN P. *Conscience and Health Care Ethics* in ASHCROFT RE ET AL (editors).*Principles of Health Care Ethics*. Hoboken: John Wiley & Sons, Ltd; 20072: 345-350.

BENJAMIN M, CURTIS J. *Ethics in Nursing: Cases, Principles, and Reasoning*. Oxford: Oxford University Press; 2010.

THE HOLY BIBLE. New American Bible Revised Edition. Washington, DC: Fairbrother; 2011: (accessed on 17.09.2014, at: http://usccb.org/bible/).

BRAMSTED K. *When Pharmacists Refuse to Dispense Prescriptions.* Lancet. 2006; 367: 1219-1220.

BRAUER K. *APhA Delegates Passed a Conscience Clause for Pharmacists* (20 April 1999). (accessed on 06.08.2014, at: http://www.gargaro.com/pharmacy/).

BROWN G. *Institutional Conscience and Catholic Health Care* in KOTERSKI JW

(editor). *Life and Learning XVI: Proceedings of the Sixteenth University Faculty for Life Conference at Villanova University.* Washington, DC: University Faculty for Life; 2007: 413-422.

BRUGGER EC. *Abortion, Conscience, and Health Care Provider Rights* (26 July 2012). Princeton; 2012 (accessed on 21.11.2014, at: http://www.thepublicdiscourse.com/2012/07/5902/).

BURKE BJ. *The Loss of a Physicians' Freedom of Conscience Will Result in the Breakdown of Patient Autonomy within the Doctor-Patient Relationship.* Linacre Q. 2009; 76 (4): 417-426.

CANADIAN NURSES ASSOCIATION. *Code of Ethics for Registered Nurses.* Ottawa: Canadian Nurses Association; 2008 (accessed on 22.11.2014, at: https://cnaaiic.ca/~/media/cna/files/en/ codeofethics.pdf).

CANTOR JD, BAUM K. *The Limits of Conscientious Objection-May Pharmacists Refuse to Fill Prescriptions for Emergency Contraception?.* N Engl J Med. 2004; 351: 2008-2012.

CANTOR JD. *Conscientious Objection Gone Awry: Restoring Selfless Professionalism in Medicine.* N Engl J Med. 2009; 360 (15): 1484-1485.

CARELESS S. *Nurses Triumphant! Human Rights Case Ends in Settlement: After a Difficult Five Year Struggle, Eight Ontario Health Care Professionals Win The Right to Choose* (May 2009). Powell River; 2009 (accessed on 26.11.2014, at: http://www.consciencelaws.org/repression/repression007.aspx).

CARRASCO DE PAOLA I, PENNACCHINI M. *Coscienza* in SGRECCIA E, TARANTINO A (editors). Enciclopedia di Bioetica e Scienza Giuridica: Vol. III Cadavere-Cyborg. Naples: Edizioni Scientifiche Italiane; 2010: 679-689.

CASAVOLA FP. *L'Obiezione di Coscienza tra Libertà e Responsabilità* in LIVERANI PG (editor). L'Obiezione di Coscienza tra Libertà e Responsabilità. Siena: Cantagalli; 2013: 19-24.

CATHOLIC NEWS AGENCY. *A 'Bullying' Move? UK Midwife Abortion Ruling Sparks Outcry* (19 December 2014). Los Angeles; 2014 (accessed on 29.12.2014, at: http://angelusnews.com/news/world/a-bullying-move-uk-midwife-abortion-rulingsparks-outcry-7115/#.VKF78c8Dk).

CAVANAUGH-O'KEEFE J. *Pro-Life Movement in the United States* in TIERNEY H (editor). *Women's Studies Encyclopedia.* Westport: Greenwood Press; 2002 (accessed on 25.11.2014, at: http://gem.greenwood.com/wse/wsePrint.jsp?id=id538).

CATHOLIC CHURCH. *Catechism of the Catholic Church* (CCC). (11 October 1992). Rome;

1992 (accessed on 17.09.2014, at: http://www.usccb.org/beliefs-andteachings/what-we-believe/ catechism/catechism-of-the-catholicchurch/epub/index.cfm#para1768).

CHADWICK H. *Betrachtungen über das Gewissen in der griechischen, jüdischen und christlichen Tradition.* Opladen:Westdeutscher Verlag; 1974.

CHAFFEE Z. *Freedom of Speech in Wartime.* Harvard Law Rev. 1919; 32: 932-973.

CHALMERS, S. *Conscience in Context: Historical and Existential Perspectives.* Bern: Peter Lang; 2013.

CHRISTIAN MEDICAL FELLOWSHIP UK. *About.* London; (accessed on 24.11.2014, at: http://www.cmf.org.uk/about/).

CHRISTIAN MEDICAL FELLOWSHIP UK. *File 39: The Doctor's Conscience.* London; 2009 (accessed on 24.08.2013, at: http://www.cmf.org.uk/publications/content.asp?context=article &id=25406).

CHRISTIAN MEDICAL FELLOWSHIP UK. *Introducing Christian Medical Fellowship.* London; (accessed on 24.11.2014, at: http://content.yudu.com/Library/A26zqv/IntroducingCMF/ resources/index.htm?referrerUrl=http%3A%2F%2Fwww.cmf.org.uk%2Fabout%2F).

CLARK BR. *When Free Exercise Exemptions Undermine Religious Liberty and the Liberty of Conscience: A Case Study of the Catholic Hospital Conflict.* Oregon Law Rev. 2013; 82 (3): 625-694.

COMBS MP, ANTIEL RM, TILBURT JC, ET AL. *Conscientious Refusals to Refer: Findings from a National Physician Survey.* J Med Ethics. 2011; 37: 397-401.

COMITATO CENTRALE DELLA FEDERAZIONE & CONSIGILIO NAZIONALE DEI COLLEGI (IPASVI). *Codice Deontologico dell'Infermiere* (2009) Rome; 2009 (accessed on 12.11.2014, at: http://www.ipasvi.it/static/ english/the-nurses-deontologicalcode-2009.htm).

COMITATO NAZIONALE PER LA BIOETICA. *Conscientious Objection and Bioethics* (30 July 2012). Rome: Presidenza del Consiglio dei Ministri, Dipartimento per l'Informazione e l'Editoria; 2012 (accessed on 11.11.2014, at: http://www.palazzochigi.it/bioetica/eng/pdf/ Conscientious_objection_bioethics_ 12_06_2012.pdf).

COMITATO NAZIONALE PER LA BIOETICA. *Note on the Pharmacist's Conscientious Objection to the Sale of Emergency Contraceptive Products* (25 February 2011). Rome; 2011 (accessed on 25.11.2014, at: http://www.governo.it/bioetica/eng/pdf/Pharmacist_ conscientious_ 20110211.pdf).

COMITATO NAZIONALE PER LA BIOETICA. *Nota sulla Contraccezione D'Emergenza* (28 May 2004). Rome: 2004 (Accessed on 18.07.2011, at; http://www.palazzochigi.it/bioetica/ testi/ contraccezione_emergenza.pdf).

COOPER WATT M. *Pharmacist Knows Best-Enacting Legislation in Oklahoma Prohibiting Pharmacists from Refusing to Provide Emergency Contraceptives.* Tulsa Law Rev. 2006; 42: 771-796.

COUNCIL OF EUROPE. *European Convention on Human Rights* (4 November 1950). Rome: Council of Europe; 1950. Art. 9. (accessed on 19.11.2014, at: http://www.echr.coe.int/ Documents/Convention_ENG.pdf).

CRANSTON M. *What are Human Rights?*. London: The Bodley Head Ltd; 1973.

CROSBY JF. *The Selfhood of the Human Person*. Washington: Catholic University of America Press; 1996.

DAAR JF. *A Clash at the Bedside: Patient Autonomy v. A Physician's Professional Conscience*. Hastings Law J. 1993; 44: 1241-1289.

DARWIN C. *The Descent of Man, and Selection in Relation to Sex*. New York: D. Appleton; 1872: Volume 1.

DAVIDSON S. *Human Rights*. Buckingham: Open University Press; 1993.

DAVIES P. *Abortion Referrals*. Triple Helix. 2010; Summer: 21 (accessed on 23.11.2014, at: http://admin.cmf.org.uk/pdf/helix/ sum10/THsum10p20-21.pdf).

DAVIS JK. *Conscientious Refusal and a Doctor's Rights to Quit*. J Med Philos. 2004; 29: 75-91.

DAWKINS R. *The God Delusion*. London: Bantam Press; 2006.

DICKENS BM, COOK RJ. *Conscientious Commitment to Women's Health*. Int J Gynaecol Obstet. 2011; 113 (2): 163-166.

DICKENS BM. *Conscientious Objection and Professionalism*. Expert Rev Obstet Gynecol. 2009; 4 (2): 97-100.

DI PIETRO ML, CASINI C, CASINI M, SPAGNOLO AG. *Obiezione di Coscienza in Sanità. Nuove Problematiche per l'Etica e per il Diritto*. Siena: Cantagalli; 2005.

DI PIETRO ML, CASINI C, CASINI M. *Obiezione di Coscienza in Sanità. Vademecum*. Siena: Cantagalli; 2009.

DI PIETRO ML, CASINI M, FIORI A, ET AL. *Norlevo e Obiezione di Coscienza*. Medicina e Morale. 2003; 53 (3): 411–455.

DONNELLY J. *International Human Rights: A Regime Analysis*. Int Organ. 1986; 40 (3): 599-642. (accessed on 28.11.2014, at: http://ernie.itpir.wm.edu/pdf/NewArticles/Liberal/2706821. pdf).

DONNELLY J. *Universal Human Rights in Theory and Practice*. Ithaca: Cornell University Press; 1989.

DUFRESNE B, MANAGAN N, MULLADY R. *Distribution of Birth Control by Pharmacists*. The Vermont Legislative Research Shop (26 April 2005) (accessed on 18.08.2014, at: https:// www.uvm. edu/~vlrs/Health/birthcontroland pharmacists.pdf).

DUNN J. *The Political Thought of John Locke: An Historical Account of the Argument of the 'Two Treatises of Government'*. Cambridge: Cambridge University Press; 1982.

DURLAND S. *The Case against Institutional Conscience*. Notre Dame Law Rev. 2011; 86 (4):

1655-1686.

DUVALL M. *Pharmacy Conscience Clause Statutes: Constitutional Religious Accommodations or Unconstitutional Substantial Burdens on Women*. American University Law Review 2005; 55; 1485-1521.

DWORKIN R. *Taking Rights Seriously*. Cambridge: Harvard University Press; 1977.

ECKEL F. *Pharmacist's Right to Choose?*. Pharmacy Times (1 July 2005). (accessed on 06.08.2014, at: http://www.pharmacytimes.com/publications/issue/2005/2005-07/2005-07-9737).

ELSHTAIN JB. *Why Science Cannot Stand Alone*. Theor Med Bioeth. 2008; 29: 161-169.

ERTELT S. LA *Nurse Wins State Supreme Court Battle in Plan B Conscience Case* (20 May 2009). Lafayette; 2009 (accessed on 26.11.2014, at: http://www.louisianamedicalnews.com/la-nurse-wins-state-supreme-court-battle-in-planb-conscience-case-cms-1309).

EUROPEAN PARLIAMENT, COUNCIL AND COMMISSION. *Charter of Fundamental Rights of the European Union* (18 December 2000). Brussels; 2000 (accessed on 22.11.2014, at: http://www.europarl.europa.eu/charter/pdf/text_en.pdf).

EUSEBI L. *L'Obiezione di Coscienza del Professionista Sanitario* in RODOTA S, ZATTI P (editors). *Trattato di Biodiritto*, Vol. III *I Diritti in Medicina*. Milan: Giuffrè; 2011: 173-187.

EXTRA DIVISION INNER HOUSE COURT OF SESSION. *Doogan & Anor v NHS Greater Glasgow & Clyde Health Board* (24 April 2013). Glasgow: ScotCS CSIH 36, appeal taken from Scot; 2013 (accessed on 19.11.2014, at: http://www.bailii.org/scot/cases/ScotCS/2013/2013CSIH36.html).

FAGAN A. *Human Rights*. Internet Encyclopedia of Philosophy, 1987. (accessed on 20.11.2014, at: http://www.iep.utm.edu/hum-rts).

FEDERAZIONI ORDINI FARMACISTI ITALIANI (FOFI). *Codice Deontologico del Farmacista* (2007). English Trans. MEANEY J. Rome; 2007 (accessed on 21.10.2014, at: http://www.fofi.it/).

FEDERAZIONE NAZIONALE DEGLI ORDINI DEI MEDICI CHIRURGHI E DEGLI ODONTOIATRI (FNOMCEO). *Codice di Deontologia Medica* (18 May 2014). English Trans. MEANEY J. Rome; 2014 (accessed on 22.11.2014, at: http://www.fnomceo.it/fnomceo/Codic e+di+Deontologia+Medica+2014. html?t=a&id=115184).

FEDORYKA D. *The Foundation of Rights in Popes John Paul II and Benedict XVI from the Perspective of the Gift*. Ave Maria Law Rev. 2012; 11 (1): 65-102.

FERGUSSON A. *Abortion Requests: Should We 'Refer'?*. Triple Helix. 2010; Easter: 14-15 (accessed on 23.11.2014, at: http://admin.cmf.org.uk/pdf/helix/spr10/th-spr10p1415.pdf).

FINNIS J. *Natural Law and Natural Rights,* Oxford: Clarendon Press; 1980.

FREEMAN M. *The Philosophical Foundations of Human Rights*. Hum Rights Q. 1994; 16: 491-514.

GAMBINO G, SPAGNOLO AG. *Ethical and Juridical Foundations of Conscientious Objection for Health Care Workers.* Med Ethika Bioet 2002; 9: 3-5.

GANS J. *Not Just a Matter of Conscience.* News Release, American Pharmacists Association (APhA) 23 June 2005.

GEDDES L. *Person.* The Catholic Encyclopedia. New York; Robert Appleton Company; 1911 (accessed on 19.11.2014, at: http://www.newadvent.org/cathen/11726a.htm).

GEISSLER H. *Conscience and Truth in the Writings of Blessed John Henry Newman.* (accessed on 04.10.2014, at: http://www.newmanfriendsinternational. org/newman/wpcontent/ uploads/2013/05/ conscience-and-truth-in-the-writings-of-blessed-jhn.pdf).

GEORGE RP. *Conscience and its Enemies: Confronting the Dogmas of Liberal Secularism.* Wilmington: ISI Books; 2013.

GEORGE RP. *Conscience and its Reviewers: A Response to Kevin Doyle* (20 November 2013). Princeton; 2013 (accessed on 17.11.2014, at: http://www.thepublicdiscourse. com/2013/11/11233/).

GERRARD JW. Is *it Ethical for a General Practitioner to Claim a Conscientious Objection When Asked to Refer for Abortion?.* J Med Ethics. 2009; 35: 599-602.

GEWIRTH A. *Reason and Morality.* Chicago: University of Chicago Press; 1978.

GOLD A. *Physicians' "Right of Conscience"-Beyond Politics.* J Law Med Ethics. 2010; 38 (1): 134-142.

GRACIA GUILLÉN D. *Fondamenti di Bioetica: Sviluppo Storico e Metodo.* Italian Trans. FELICIANI AJ, SPINSANTI S. Milan: Edizioni San Paolo; 1993.

GRADY A. *Legal Protection for Conscientious Objection by Health Professionals.* Virtual Mentor. 2006; 8 (5): 327-331.

GRIFFIN J. On Human Rights. Oxford: Oxford University Press; 2013.

HAAS J. *Crisis of Conscience and Culture* in HAAS J (editor). *Crisis of Culture.* New York: Crossroad; 1996: 21-47.

HARDT JJ. *The Conscience Debate: Resources for Rapprochement from the Problem's Perceived Source.* TheorMed Bioeth. 2008; 29: 151-160.

HARE RD. *Without Conscience: The Disturbing World of the Psychopaths Among Us.* New York: Guilford Press; 1999.

HARRIS LH. *Recognizing Conscience in Abortion Provision.* N Engl J Med. 2012; 367 (11): 981-983.

HEANEY SJ. *Protecting Conscience in Health Care: Taking a Road Not Travelled.* Natl Cathol Bioeth Q. 2008; 8 (4): 673-680.

HEINO A, GISSLER M, APTER D, ET AL. *Conscientious Objection and Induced Abortion in Europe.* Eur J Contracep Reprod Health Care. 2013; 18: 231-233.

HOGAN L. *Confronting the Truth: Conscience in the Catholic Tradition.* Mahwah: Paulist

Press; 2000.

HOOKER B. *On Human Rights* [Book Review]. Oxf J Leg Stud. 2010; 30 (1): 193-205.

IGLESIAS ROZAS T. *Newman on Conscience and our Culture.* Milltown Studies. 2002; 49: 19-49.

IMBODY J. *Data and Analysis of Two National Surveys on Conscience Rights Regulation and Laws, as Related to HHS Requested Information on Rescission Proposal.* (9 April 2009). Bristol; 2009 (accessed on 24.11.2014, at: http://cmda.org/library/doclib/cma-survey-analysis-for-hhs.pdf).

INTERNATIONAL CONFERENCE ON HUMAN RIGHTS. *Proclamation of Teheran* (13 May 1968). Teheran; 1968 (accessed on 09.28.2014, at: http://www1.umn.edu/humanrts/ instree/ l2ptichr.htm).

ITALIAN CONSTITUTIONAL COURT. *Sentenza N. 467* (16 December 1991). English Trans. Meaney J. Rome; 1991 (accessed on 18.07.2011, at:http://www.cortecostituzionale.it/ action Pronuncia.do).

ITALIAN PARLIAMENT. *Legge 22 maggio 1978, n. 194 Norme per la Tutela Sociale della Maternità e sull'Interruzione Volontaria della Gravidanza* (22 May 1978). Rome; 1978 (accessed on 18.08.2014, at: http://www.salute.gov.it/imgs/C_17_normativa_845_allegato.pdf).

ITALIAN REPUBLIC. *Constitution of the Republic of Italy* (22 December 1947). Rome; 1947 (accessed on 21.11.2014, at: https://www.senato.it/documenti/repository/istituzione/ costituzione _inglese.pdf).

JAGER E. *The Book of the Heart.* Chicago: University of Chicago Press; 2000.

JANSEN L. *HIV Exceptionalism, CD4+ Cell Testing, and Conscientious Subversion.* J Med Ethics. 2005; 31 (6): 322-326.

JOHN XXIII. *Pacem in Terris.* (11 April 1963). Rome; 1963 (accessed on 20.11.2014, at: http:// www. vatican.va/holy_father/john_xxiii/encyclicals/documents/hf_j-xxiii_enc_11041963_ pacem_en. html).

JOHN PAUL II. *Evangelium Vitae.* (25 March 1995). Rome; 1995 (accessed on 25.11.2014, at: http://www.vatican.va/holy_father/john_paul_ii/encyclicals/documents/hf_jp-ii_ enc_25031995_evangelium-vitae_en.html).

JOHN PAUL II. *Veritatis Splendor.* (6 August 1993). Rome; 1993 (accessed on 18.09.2014, at: http://www.vatican.va/holy_father/john_paul_ii/encyclicals/documents/hf_jp-ii_ enc_06081993_ veritatis-splendor_en.html).

JONSEN AR, SIEGLER M, WINSLADE WJ. *Un Approccio Pratico alle Decisioni Etiche in Medicina Clinica.* Italian Trans. FALLANI A. SPAGNOLO AG (editor). Milan: The McGraw Hill Companies, Inc.; 2003.

JONES C. *Druggists Refuse to Give Out Pill.* USA Today. (9 November 2004). Tyson's Corner; 2004 (accessed on 20.08.2014, at: http://usatoday30.usatoday.com/news/nation/2004-11-08-

druggists-pill_ x.htm).

KACZOR K. *Abortion, Conscience, and Doctors* (29 October 2010). Princeton; 2010 (accessed on 24.11.2014, at: http://www.thepublicdiscourse.com/2010/10/1922/).

KANT I. Kant: *Groundwork of the Metaphysics of Morals*. English Trans. GREGOR MJ. Cambridge: Cambridge University Press. 1998.

KANTYMIR L, MCLEOD C. *Justification for Conscience Exemptions in Health Care*. Bioethics. 2014; 28 (1): 16-23.

KING ML Jr. *Letter from Birmingham Jail* (16 April 1963) Birmingham: 1963 (accessed on 21.10.2014, at: http://www.africa.upenn.edu/Articles_Gen/Letter_Birmingham.html).

KISKA R. *Sweden's Aggressive Attack on Conscience Challenged Before the Council of Europe*. Zenit (14 June 2014). Rome; 2014 (accessed on 19.11.2014, at: http://www.zenit.org/en/articles/sweden-s-aggressive-attack-on-conscience-challengedbefore-the-council-of-europe).

KLEIN E. *Establishing a Hierarchy of Human Rights: Ideal Solution or Fallacy?*. Isr Law Rev. 2008; 41: 477-488.

KNESSET OF THE STATE OF ISRAEL. *Criminal Law Amendment (Interruption of Pregnancy) Law*. Jerusalem: Knesset; 1977: (accessed on 18.07.2011, at: http://www.hsph.harvard.edu/population/abortion/ISRAEL.abo.htm).

KNIGHT BIXLER G, WHITE BIXLER R. *The Professional Status of Nursing*. Am J Nurs. 1945; 45 (9): 730-735.

KNOWLEDGE BASE. *What is a Normal Survey Response Rate?*. (accessed on 22.11.2014, at: http://support2.constantcontact.com/articles/FAQ/2344).

KOJI T. *Emerging Hierarchy in International Human Rights and Beyond: From the Perspective of Non-Derogable Rights*, Eur J Int Law. 2001; 12: 917-941.

KORBE T. *Court: New Jersey Nurses Don't Have to Assist With Abortions* (23 December 2011). Washington DC; 2011 (accessed on 26.11.2014, at: http://hotair.com/archives/2011/12/23court-new-jersey-nurses-dont-have-to-assist-with-abortions/).

KOSKENNIEMI M. *Hierarchy in International Law: A Sketch*. Eur J Int Law. 1997; 8: 566-582.

KUBALA MT. *Obieziene di Coscienza e Rivendicazione Abortista in Europa* [dissertation]. Rome: Pontifical University of the Holy Cross; 2013.

LACLAU, E. & MOUFFE, C. Hegemony and Socialist Strategy. English Trans. MOORE W, COMMACK P. New York: Verso; 1985.

LAFFITTE J. *Storia dell'Obiezione di Coscienza e Differenti Accezioni del Concetto di Tolleranza* in SGRECCIA E, LAFFITTE J (editors). *La Coscienza Christiana a Sostegno del Diritto alla Vita*. Rome: Libreria Editrice Vaticana; 2008: 112-139.

LATKOVIC MS. *Pro-Life Nurses and Cooperation in Abortion: Ordinary Care or Extraordinary Intervention?*. Natl Cathol Bioeth Q. 2004; 4 (1): 89-102.

LAMACKOVÁ A. *Conscientious Objection in Reproductive Health Care: Analysis of Pichon and Sajous v. France.* Eur J Health Law. 2008; 15 (1): 7-43.

LANGSTON DC. *Conscience and Other Virtues: From Bonaventure to MacIntyre.* University Park: Penn State Press; 2008.

LASSI ZS, COMETTO G, HUICHO L, ET AL. *Quality of Care Provided by Mid-Level Health Workers: Systematic Review and Meta-Analysis.* Bull World Health Organ. 2013; 91: 824-833. p. 24. [On-line journal]. (accessed on 20.11.2014 at: http://www.who.int/bulletin/volumes/91/11/13-118786.pdf).

LAWRENCE RE, CURLIN FA. *Clash of Definitions: Controversies About Conscience in Medicine.* Am J Bioeth. 2007; 7 (12): 10-14.

LAWRENCE RE, CURLIN FA. *Physicians' Beliefs About Conscience in Medicine: A National Survey.* Acad Med. 2009; 84 (9): 1276-1282.

LEWIN T. *Rights of Citizens and Society Raise Legal Muddle on AIDS.* New York Times (14 October 1987) New York; 1987.

LEWIS CS. *The Abolition of Man.* New York: Harper Collins; 2001.

LEWIS CS. *Mere Christianity.* London: Collins; 1988.

LINEWEAVER CH. *Increasingly Overlapping Magisteria of Science and Religion* in GORDON R, SECKBACH J (editors). *Divine Action and Natural Selection: Questions of Science and Faith in Biological Evolution.* Singapore:World Scientific; 2008: 171-181.

LIVERANI PG. *Coscienza o Autodeterminazione?* in LIVERANI PG (editor). *L'Obiezione di Coscienza tra Libertà e Responsabilità.* Siena: Cantagalli; 2013: 119-121.

LOCKE J. *A Letter Concerning Toleration.* Minneapolis: Filiquarian Publishing LLC; 2007.

MACINTYRE A. *After Virtue: A Study in Moral Theory.* London: Duckworth; 1981.

MARITAIN J. *The Rights of Man and Natural Law.* London: The Centenary Press; 1945.

MARTIN DE AGAR JT. *Problemas Jurídicos de la Objeción de Conciencia.* ScriptaTheologica. 1995; 2: 519-543.

MAY T, AULISIO MP. *Personal Morality and Professional Obligations. Right of Conscience and Informed Consent.* Perspect Biol Med 2009; 52: 30-38.

MCCAFFERTY C. *Women's Access to Lawful Medical Care: The Problem of the Unregulated Use of Conscientious Objection* (10 July 2010) Strasbourg; 2010 (accessed on 19.11.2014, at: http://assembly.coe.int/ASP/Doc/XrefViewPDF.asp?FileID=12506&Language=EN).

MEANEY J. *É un Bene per i Pazienti l'Obiezione di Coscienza del Medico?.* Medicina e Morale. 2011; 60 (5): 930-933.

MEANEY J, CASINI M, SPAGNOLO AG. *Objective Reason for Conscientious Objection in Health Care.* Natl Cathol Bioeth Q. 2012; 12 (4): 611-620.

MEIRON THOMAS J. *Why Having so Many Women Doctors is Hurting the NHS: A Provocative but Powerful Argument from a Leading Surgeon.* Mail Online (2 January 2014). London; 2014 (accessed on 24.11.2014, at: http://www.dailymail.co.uk/debate/article-2532461/Why-having-women-doctors-hurting-NHS-A-provovcative-powerfulargument-leading-surgeon.html).

MERGER WATCH. *In Medical Care, the Patients Rights Must Come First.* New York; 2014 (accessed on 30.10.2014, at: http://www.mergerwatch.org/about/).

MILL JS. *On Liberty.* London: Longmans, Green, and Company; 1921:

MORE T. *Letter to Margaret Roper from the Tower of London* (June 3, 1535). London; 1535 (accessed on 25.10.2014, at: http://www.thomasmorestudies.org/quotes.html).

NAIRN TA. *Institutional Conscience Revisited Catholic Institutions and Christian Ethics.* New Theol Rev. 2001; 14: 39-49.

NATIONAL ASSOCIATION OF BOARDS OF PHARMACY (NABP). *Conscience Clause Controversy on Back Burner, but Still Simmering.* NABP Newsletter, 22 April 2011 (accessed on 20.08.2014, at: http://www.nabp.net/news/conscience-clausecontroversy-on-back-burner-but-still-simmering/).

NATIONAL CONFERENCE OF STATE LEGISLATURES (NCSL) HEALTH PROGRAM. *Pharmacist Conscience Clauses: Laws and Information* (May 2012). Denver; 2012 (accessed on 20.08.2014, at: http://www.ncsl.org/research/health/pharmacist-conscience-clauses-laws-and-information.aspx).

NEWMAN JH. *An Essay in Aid of a Grammar of Assent.* KER I. (editor). Oxford: Clarendon Press; 1985.

NEWMAN JH. *Dispositions for Faith.* sermon no 5 in *Sermons Preached on Various Occasions.* London: Longmans, Green, and Co.; 1908: p. 60-74. (accessed on 21.11.2014, at: http://www.newmanreader.org/works/occasions/).

NEWMAN JH. *Sermon Notes.* Notre Dame: University of Notre Dame Press; 2000.

NEWMAN JH. *Sermons Preached on Various Occasions.* London: Longmans, Green, and Co.; 1908: (accessed on 21.11.2014, at: http://www.newmanreader.org/works/occasions/).

NIETZSCHE F. *On the Genealogy of Morals: A Polemical Tract.* English Trans. JOHNSTON I. Arlington: Richer Resources Publications; 2009 (accessed on 17.11.2014, at: http://home.sandiego.edu/~janderso/360/genealogy2.htm).

NICKEL J. *Making Sense of Human Rights: Philosophical Reflections on the Universal Declaration of Human Rights.* Berkeley: University of California Press; 1987.

OFFICE OF THE UNITED NATIONS HIGH COMMISSIONER FOR HUMAN RIGHTS (OHCHR). *Frequently Asked Questions on a Human Rights-Based Approach to Development Cooperation.* New York: OHCR; 2006 (accessed on 19.11.2014, at: http://www.ohchr.org/Documents/Publications/FAQen.pdf).

OUTER HOUSE COURT OF SESSION. *Doogan & Anor v NHS Greater Glasgow & Clyde Health Board* (29 February 2012). Glasgow: ScotCS CSIH 32, appeal taken from Scot; 2012 (accessed on 19.11.2014, at: http://www.scotcourts.gov.uk/opinions/ 2012CSOH32.html).

PARLIAMENTARY ASSEMBLY OF THE COUNCIL OF EUROPE. *Recommendation 1518 (2001): Exercise of the Right of Conscientious Objection to Military Service in Council of Europe Member States* (23 May 2001). Strasbourg; 2001 (accessed on 22.11.2014, at: http://www. refworld.org/docid/5107cf8f2.html).

PARLIAMENTARY ASSEMBLY OF THE COUNCIL OF EUROPE. *Resolution 1763 The Right to Conscientious Objection in Lawful Medical Care* (7 October 2010). Strasbourg; 2010 (accessed on 19.11.2014, at: http://assembly.coe.int/Mainf.asp?link=/Documents/ AdoptedText/ta10/ ERES1763.htm).

PARLIAMENTARY ASSEMBLY OF THE COUNCIL OF EUROPE COMMITTEE ON EQUAL OPPORTUNITIES FOR WOMEN AND MEN. *Committee Opinion Doc. 12389* (6 October 2010) Strasbourg; 2010 (accessed on 18.07.2011, at: http://assembly.coe.int/Main. asp?link=/Documents/WorkingDocs/ Doc10/ EDOC12389.htm).

PARLIAMENTARY COUNCIL OF THE FEDERAL REPUBLIC OF GERMANY. *Basic Law for the Federal Republic of Germany*. Berlin: Federal Law Gazette; 1990: (accessed on 18.07.2011, at: http://www. constitution.org/cons/germany.txt).

PARLIAMENTARY NETWORK FOR CRITICAL ISSUES. *Georgetown Law Entity Co-Authors Document Targeting Conscientious Objection*. Parliamentary Network ENews. 2014; 8 (10): November 2014 (accessed on 29.11.2014, at: http://www.pncius.org/index.aspx).

PAUL VI. *Declaration on Religious Freedom: Dignitatis Humanae*. (7 December 1965). Rome; 1965 (accessed 17.09.2014, at: http://www.vatican.va/archive/hist_councils/ii_vatican_ council/ documents/vat-ii_decl_19651207_dignitatis-humanae_en.html).

PAUL VI. *Pastoral Constitution on the Church in the Modern World: Gaudium et Spes*. (7 December 1965). Rome; 1965 (accessed 17.09.2014, at: http://www.vatican.va/archive/ hist_ councils/ii_vatican_council/documents/vat-ii_cons_19651207_gaudium-etspes_en.html).

PAVONE G. *Medici Obiettori: Un Problema Italiano*. La Repubblica (17 November 2011). Rome; 2011 (accessed on 08.10.2014, at: http://d.repubblica.it/argomenti/2011/11/17/news/ medici_ obiettori-668839/).

PELLEGRINO ED. *Engaging the Whole Breadth of Reason: Catholic Bioethics in the University and in the Post-Secular World* in KOTERSKI JW (editor). *Life and Learning XVIII: Proceedings of the Eighteenth University Faculty for Life Conference*. Bronx: University Faculty for Life; 2011: 3-19.

PELLEGRINO ED. *La Conciencia del Medico, Cláusulas de Conciencia y Creencia Religiosa: una Perspectiva Católica*. Spanish Trans. SANTIAGO M. Cuadernos de Bioética 2014; 25 (3): 25-40.

PELLEGRINO ED. *The Medical Profession as a Moral Community*. Bull NY Acad Med. 1990;

66 (3): 221-232.

PELLEGRINO ED. *Patient and Physician Autonomy: Conflicting Rights and Obligations in the Physician-Patient Relationship.* J Contemp Health Law Policy.1994; 10: 47-68.

PELLEGRINO ED. *Societal Duty and Moral Complicity: The Physician's Dilemma of Divided Loyalty.* Int J Law Psychiatry. 1993; 16: 371-391.

PERRY MJ. *The Idea of Human Rights: Four Inquiries.* Oxford: Oxford University Press; 2000.

PIERCE CA. *Conscience in the New Testament.* London: SCM Press; 1955.

PILLAY N. *Statement by Navi Pillay, the UN High Commissioner for Human Rights at the Deposit of the 10th Ratification Instrument, by Uruguay, of the Optional Protocol of the International Covenant on Economic, Social and Cultural Rights, Delivered by Assistant Secretary-General for Human Rights Ivan Šimonović* (6 February 2013). New York; 2013 (accessed on 20.11.2014, at: http://www.ohchr.org/EN/NewsEvents/Pages/DisplayNews. aspx?NewsID= 12971&LangID=E).

PLATO. *Apology.* English Trans. JOWETT B. Salt Lake City: Project Gutenberg Literary Archive Foundation; 2008 (accessed on 20.11.2014, at: http://www.gutenberg.org/files/1656/1656-h/1656-h.htm).

PLATO. *Plato's Gorgias.* English Trans. JOWETT B. Rockville, Maryland: Serenity Publishers LLC; 2009.

PRZETACZNIK F. *The Right to Life as a Basic Human Right.* Hum Rights J. 1976; 9: 589-603.

QUEENSLAND PUBLIC INTEREST LAW CLEARING HOUSE INC. (QPILCH). *The Hierarchy of Human Rights.* QPILCH Database, Brisbane (accessed on 28.09.2014, at: http://www.qpilch.org.au/_dbase_upl/E_Human Rights.pdf).

RATZINGER J. *On Conscience.* San Francisco: Ignatius Press; 2007.

REQUENA P. *Un Paradosso della Bioetica Nordamericana: Autonomia vs. Conscienza.* Acta Philosophica. 2011; 20 (1): 167-171.

REVERBY SM. *More Than Fact and Fiction: Cultural Memory and the Tuskegee Syphilis Study.* Hastings Cent Rep. 2001; 31 (5): 22-28.

RICO B. *Los Médicos Emprenden Acciones Contra el Nuevo Código Ético Profesional.* Granada Hoy (3 July 2011). Granada; 2011 (accessed on 18.07.2011, at: http://www.granadahoy.com/article/granada/1012493/los/medicos/emprenden/acciones/contra/nuevo/codigo/etico/profesional.html).

ROUSSE ST. *Professional Autonomy in Medicine: Defending the Right of Conscience in Health Care Beyond the Right to Religious Freedom.* Linacre Q. 2012; 79 (2): 155-168.

RORTY R. *Contingency, Irony and Solidarity.* Cambridge: Cambridge University Press; 1989.

SACCHINI D, ANTICO L. *The Professional Autonomy of the Medical Doctor in Italy.* Theor Med Bioeth. 2000; 21 (5): 441-456.

SÁEZ CABRERA C. *La Desobedencia Civil. Anuario de Derechos Humanos*. Nueva Época. 2000; 1: 311-355.

SAUNDERS P. *Freedom of Conscience in Medicine is Under Sustained Attack but is Worth Fighting for* (16 June 2014). London; 2014 (accessed on 22.11.2014, at: http://pjsaunders. blogspot.it/2014/ 06/freedom-of-conscience-in-medicine-is.html).

SAUNDERS W, SMITH M. *Pro-Life Pharmacists Win Huge Victory in Illinois Decision*. LifeNews. com, 24 September 2012 (accessed 20.08.2014, at: http://www.lifenews.com/2012/09/24/pro-life-pharmacists-win-huge-victory-in-illinois-decision/).

SAVITA S, GANDHI M, GANDHI S, ET AL. *Satyagraha*. New Delhi: Publications Division, Indian Ministry of Information and Broadcasting; 2007.

SAVULESCU J. *Conscientious Objection in Medicine*. Br Med J. 2006; 332: 294-297.

SCHELER M. *Reue und Wiedergeburt* in SCHELER M (editor). *Vom Ewigen im Menschen*. Bern/Munich: Francke-Verlag; 1968: 27-59.

SCOFIELD M. *T.S. Eliot: The Poems*. Cambridge: Cambridge University Press; 1988.

SEIFERT J. *Is the Right to Life or Is Another Right the Most Fundamental Human Right – The 'Urgrundrecht'?: Human Dignity, Moral Obligations, Natural Rights and Positive Law*. J East-West Thought. 2013; 3 (4): 11-31. (accessed on 19.11.2014, at: http://www.csupomona. edu/~jet/ Documents/JET/Jet9/Seifert11-31.pdf).

SEIFERT J. *Philosophische Grundlagen der Menschenrechte: Zur Verteidigung des Menschen*. Prima Philosophia 5/4 (1988): 339-370.

SEPPER E. *Taking Conscience Seriously*. Virginia Law Rev. 2012; 98: 1501-1575.

SEN A. *Development as Freedom*. Oxford: Oxford University Press; 1999.

SGRECCIA E. *Personalist Bioethics Foundations and Applications*. English Trans. DI CAMILLO JA, MILLER MJ. Philadelphia: National Catholic Bioethics Center; 2012.

SHELTON D. *Hierarchy of Norms and Human Rights: Of Trumps and Winners*. Sask Law Rev. 2002; 65: 301-331

SHESTACK JJ. *The Philosophical Foundations of Human Rights*. Hum Rts Q. 20 (1998), 201-234.

SMITH J. *Protecting the Careers of Medical Professionals Who Believe in the Hippocratic Oath* (27 May 2009). Powell River; 2009 (accessed on 12.11.2014, at: http://www.consciencelaws. org/ issues-legal/legal048.html).

SNYDER L. *American College of Physicians Ethics Manual: Sixth Edition*. Ann Intern Med. 2012; 156 (1_Part_2): 73-104.

SOPHOCLES. *Antigone; Oedipus the King; Electra*. English Trans. DAVY H, KITTO F. Oxford: Oxford University Press; 1994.

STROHM P. *Conscience: A Very Short Introduction*. Oxford: Oxford University Press; 2011.

SUADEAU J. *L'Objection de Conscience ou le Devoir de Désobéir.* Valence: Editions Peuple Libre; 2013.

SULMASSY DP. *What is Conscience and Why is Respect for it so Important?* Theor Med Bioeth. 2008; 29: 135-149.

SUPREME COURT OF THE UNITED KINGDOM. *Greater Glasgow Health Board (Appellant) v Doogan and another (Respondents) (Scotland)* (17 December 2014). London; 2014: §11 (accessed on 29.12.2014, at: https://www.supremecourt.uk/decidedcases/docs/ UKSC_2013_0124_ Judgment.pdf).

SWEDISH PARLIAMENT. *Freedom of Conscience in Health Care* (11 May 2011). Stockholm; 2011 (accessed on 19.11.2014, at: http://www.consciencelaws.org/background/society/society 004.aspx).

TAYLOR PE. *From Environmental to Ecological Human Rights: A New Dynamic in International Law?.* Georget Int Environ Law Rev. 10 (1997): 309-397.

TAYLOR T. *Opening Statement in the Doctors Trial.* (9 December 1946). Nuremberg; 1946 (accessed on 19.09.2014, at: http://law2.umkc.edu/faculty/projects/ftrials/nurembergdoctoropen. html).

THOMASMA DC. *Beyond Medical Paternalism and Patient Autonomy: A Model of Physician Conscience for the Physician-Patient Relationship.* Ann Intern Med. 1983; 98 (2): 243-248.

THOREAU HD. *Civil Disobedience.* (Original Title: Resistance to Civil Government) Concord; 1849 (accessed on 20.10.2014, at: http://www.transcendentalists.com/civil_disobedience. htm).

TOLLEFSEN CO. *An Absolute Liberty of Conscience?* (9 January 2009). Princeton; 2009 (accessed on 23.11.2014, at: http://www.thepublicdiscourse.com/2009/01/100/).

TOLLEFSEN CO. *Protecting Positive Claims of Conscience for Employees of Religious Institutions Threatens Religious Liberty.* Virtual Mentor. 2013; 15 (3) 236-239.

TURCHI V. *I Nuovi Volti di Antigone. Le Obiezioni di Coscienza nell'Esperienza Giuridica Contemporanea.* Naples: ESI; 2009.

TURCHI V. *Nuove Forme di Obiezione di Coscienza. Stato, Chiese e Pluralismo Confessionale.* (October 2010). Milan; 2010 (accessed on 18.11.2014, at: http://www.statoechiese.it/images/ stories/2010.10/turchi_ nuove.pdf).

TWOMEY DV. *Pope Benedict XVI: The Conscience of Our Age A Theological Portrait.* San Francisco: Ignatius Press; 2007.

UNITED NATIONS COMMITTEE ON ECONOMIC, SOCIAL AND CULTURAL RIGHTS. *Fact Sheet No.16,* (REV.1). New York: OHCHR. 1991 (accessed on 21.11.2014, at: http://www. ohchr. org/Documents/Publications/FactSheet16rev.1en.pdf).

UNITED STATES DEPARTMENT OF HEALTH AND HUMAN SERVICES (HHS).

Regulation for the Enforcement of Federal Health Care Provider Conscience Protection Laws

(23 February 2011). Washington DC; 2011(accessed on 11.11.2014, at: http://edocket.access. gpo.gov/2011/pdf/ 2011-3993.pdf).

UNITED NATIONS GENERAL ASSEMBLY. *Charter of the United Nations* (26 June 1945). San Francisco; 1945 (accessed on 09.10.2014, at: https://www.un.org/en/documents/charter/ chapter9. shtml).

UNITED NATIONS GENERAL ASSEMBLY. *International Covenant on Civil and Political Rights* (23 March 1976). New York; 1976 (accessed on 19.09.2014, at: http://www.ohchr.org/ EN/ ProfessionalInterest/Pages/CCPR.aspx).

UNITED NATIONS GENERAL ASSEMBLY. *Universal Declaration of Human Rights* (10 December 1948). Paris; 1948 (accessed on 19.09.2014, at: http://www.un.org/en/documents/ udhr/index.shtml#a18).

UNITED NATIONS HUMAN RIGHTS OFFICE OF THE HIGH COMMISSIONER. *Vienna Declaration and Programme of Action*: 20 Years Working for Your Rights 1993 World Conference on Human Rights. New York: OHCHR and the United Nations Department of Public Information. 2013 (accessed on 21.11.2014, at: http://www.ohchr.org/Documents/ Events/OHCHR20/VDPA _booklet_English.pdf).

UNITED NATIONS INTERNATIONAL LAW COMMISSION. *Principles of International Law Recognized in the Charter of the Nürnberg Tribunal and in the Judgment of the Tribunal.* (29 July 1950). Geneva; 1950 (accessed on 19.09.2014, at: http://legal.un.org/ilc/texts/ instruments/english/ draft%20articles/7_1_1950.pdf).

UNITED STATES CONFERENCE OF CATHOLIC BISHOPS. *Ethical and Religious Directives for Catholic Health Care Services* (17 November 2009). Washington DC; 20095 (accessed on 30.10.2014, at: http://www.usccb.org/issues-and-action/human-lifeand-dignity/health-care/ upload/Ethical-Religious-Directives-Catholic-Health-Care-Services-fifth-edition-2009. pdf).

UNITED STATES DEPARTMENT OF HEALTH AND HUMAN SERVICES (HHS). *Regulation for the Enforcement of Federal Health Care Provider Conscience Protection Laws* (23 February 2011). Washington DC; 2011(accessed on 11.11.2014, at: http://edocket.access. gpo.gov/2011/ pdf/2011-3993.pdf).

VACCA MA. *A Reexamination of Conscience Protections in Healthcare.* Medicina e Morale. 2013; 62 (6): 1203-1207.

VELEZ JR. *Freedom of Conscience in Ethical Decision Making.* Linacre Q. 2009; 76 (2): 120-132.

VIOLA F. *L'Obiezione di Coscienza Come Diritto.* Persona y Derecho. 2009; 61: 53-71.

VISCHER RK. *Conscience and the Common Good: Reclaiming the Space Between Person and the State.* Cambridge: Cambridge University Press; 2010.

WALL LL, BROWN D. *Refusals by Pharmacists to Dispense Emergency Contraception: A Critique.* Obstet Gynecol 2006; 107: 1148-1151.

WARDLE LD. *Protection of Health-Care Providers' Rights of Conscience in American Law*: Present, Past, and Future. Ave Maria Law Rev. 2010. 9 (1): 1-46.

WARDLE LD. *Rights of Conscience vs. Peer-Driven Medical Ethics: ACOG and Abortion* in KOTERSKI JW (editor). Life and Learning XVIII: Proceedings of the Eighteenth University Faculty for Life Conference. Bronx: University Faculty for Life; 2011: 23-56.

WEBER E. *Positive and Negative Rights: What's the Difference, and Why Does It Matter?* (2May 2009). San Francisco; 2009 (accessed on 27.08.2014, at: http://everydayethics.org/positive-and-negative-rights-whats-the-difference-and-why-does-it-matter/).

WEBER T. *Gandhi as Disciple and Mentor*. Cambridge: Cambridge University Press; 2004.

WEIL S. *Dieu dans Platon* in CAMUS A. (editor). La Source Grecque. Paris: Gallimard; 1953; 5: 67-126.

WEIL S. *OEuvres complètes V, 2: Écrits de New York et de Londres* (1943). Paris: Gallimard; 2013.

WELLMAN C. *Solidarity, the Individual and Human Rights*. Hum Rights Q. 2000; 22: 639-657.

WERNER B. *Affidavit*. (18 February 1947). Nuremberg; 1947 (accessed on 19.09.2014, at: http://nuremberg.law.harvard.edu/php/pflip.php?caseid=HLSL_NMT01&docnum=347&numpages=2&startpage=1&title=Affidavit..&color_setting=C).

WHITE DB, BRODY B. *Would Accommodating Some Conscientious Objections by Physicians Promote Quality in Medical Care?*. JAMA. 2011; 305 (17): 1804-1805.

WICCLAIR MR. *Conscientious Objection in Health Care an Ethical Analysis*. Cambridge: Cambridge University Press; 2011.

WICCLAIR MR. *Conscientious Objection in Medicine*. Bioethics. 2000; 14 (3): 205-227.

WICCLAIR MR. *Is Conscientious Objection Incompatible with a Physician's Professional Obligations?* TheorMed Bioeth. 2008; 29: 171-185.

WICCLAIR MR. *Negative and Positive Claims of Conscience*. Camb Q Healthc Ethics. 2009; 18: 14-22.

WIKE B. *Darwin and the Descent of Morality*. First Things. 2001; 12 (9): (accessed on 17.11.2014, at: http://www.firstthings.com/article/2001/11/darwin-and-the-descentof morality).

WILLIAMS TD. *Who Is My Neighbor? Personalism and the Foundations of Human Rights*. Washington DC: Catholic University of America Press: 2005.

WOJTYLA K. *The Acting Person*. English Trans. POTOCKI A. Dordrecht: Reidel; 1979.

WOLFF R. *Conscientious Objection: Time for Recognition as a Fundamental Human Right*. ASILS Int Law J. 1982; 6: 65-95.

WOMEN'S LINK WORLDWIDE. *Balancing Conscience and Women's Reproductive Rights* (24 October 2014). Madrid; 2014 (accessed 18.11.2014, at: http://www.womenslinkworldwide. org/ wlw/new. php?modo=detalle_prensa&dc=469).

WORLD CONFERENCE ON HUMAN RIGHTS. *Vienna Declaration and Programme of Action* (25 June 1993). Vienna; 1993 (accessed on 21.11.2014, at: http://www.ohchr.org/Documents/ProfessionalInterest/vienna.pdf).

WORLD HEALTH ORGANIZATION. *Health Topics: Midwifery.* (accessed on 19.11.2014, at: http://www.who.int/topics/midwifery/en/).

WORLD MEDICAL ASSOCIATION (WMA). *Physician's Oath* (September 1948). Geneva; 1948 (accessed on 18.07.2011, at: http://www.mma.org.my/Portals/0/Declaration%20of%20Geneva.pdf).

WRIGHT M. *Euripides: Orestes.* London: Gerald Duckworth & Co. Ltd.; 2008.

XIAOBING X, WILSON G. *On Conflict of Human Rights.* Pierce Law Rev. 2006; 5 (1):31-57.

Joseph Meaney, PhD

Dr. Joseph Meaney is the director of international outreach and expansion at Human Life International. One of the world's leading experts on the international pro-life movement, Dr. Joseph Meaney speaks French, Spanish, and Italian fluently.

He is the son of Drs. Michael and Francette Meaney. Joseph was born and raised in Corpus Christi, Texas where he attended St. Patrick's Catholic School, Bishop Garriga Junior High and Incarnate Word Academy.

His bachelors and masters degrees from the University of Dallas and the University of Texas Institute of Latin American Studies prepared him for an international career that has included lectures and investigative journalism missions on all continents and over 74 countries. Joseph completed in 2015 his PhD in Bioethics at the Catholic University of the Sacred Heart in Rome. He currently works out of the new HLI office in Paris, France, where he resides with his wife, Marie and their daughter, Thérèse.

Joseph's work has been featured in publications such as The American Spectator, Crisis Magazine, Inside Catholic, National Catholic Bioethics Quarterly, LifeSiteNews, and the National Catholic Register. He was the general editor of the English edition of Lexicon: Ambiguous and Debatable Terms Regarding Family Life and Ethical Questions, published by Human Life International, 2006. He also appeared in the pro-life documentary "Silent Fall," and is featured in HLI's documentaries which debuted on EWTN "Central and Eastern Europe: A Return to Life" and "Central America and Mexico: Fighting for Life, Faith and Family."